SEEKING SICKNESS

FOREWORD BY **DR.H.GILBERT WELCH**

SEEKING SICKNESS

Medical Screening and the Misguided Hunt for Disease

ALAN CASSELS

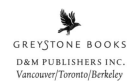

GREYSTONE BOOKS

D&M PUBLISHERS INC.

Vancouver/Toronto/Berkeley

Greystone Books
An imprint of D&M Publishers Inc.
2323 Quebec Street, Suite 201
Vancouver BC Canada V5T 4S7
www.greystonebooks.com

Cataloguing data available from Library and Archives Canada
ISBN 978-1-77100-032-1 (pbk.)
ISBN 978-1-77100-033-8 (ebook)

Editing by Catherine Plear
Cover design by Setareh Ashrafologhalai
Text design by Naomi MacDougall
Cover photograph © Chris Whitehead/Getty Images
Printed and bound in Canada by Friesens
Distributed in the U.S. by Publishers Group West

Some of this material was previously published
in a different form in *Common Ground, The Tyee,* and
the *Canadian Medical Association Journal.*

We gratefully acknowledge the financial support of the Canada
Council for the Arts, the British Columbia Arts Council, the Province
of British Columbia through the Book Publishing Tax Credit,
and the Government of Canada through the Canada
Book Fund for our publishing activities.

Greystone Books is committed to reducing the
consumption of old-growth forests in the books it publishes.
This book is one step towards that goal.

For Earle Cassels

CONTENTS

THE LAST fifty years have seen dramatic changes in medical care. Many have translated into real improvements for patients—most notably for those are who genuinely sick, for whom diagnoses are now both more prompt and more accurate and for whom treatments are now both more effective and less morbid.

But not all of the changes in medical care represent real improvement. Many have produced much more mixed effects: perhaps helping some, but also hurting others.

Case in point: Fifty years ago, doctors made diagnoses and initiated therapy only in patients who were experiencing problems. Of course, we doctors still do that today. But increasingly we also operate under a new paradigm: seeking diagnosis and initiating therapy in people who are *not* experiencing problems. That's a huge change in paradigms, from one that focused on the sick to one that focuses on the well.

Think about it this way: In the past, you went to the doctor because you had a problem and you wanted to learn what to do about it. Now you go to the doctor because you want to stay well and you learn instead that you have a problem.

The new paradigm is early diagnosis. It goes something like this: The best way to keep people healthy is to find (pick one) heart disease, autism, glaucoma, vascular problems, osteoporosis, or any cancer early. And the way to find these conditions early is through screening.

But the medical profession is just beginning to understand the downside of early diagnosis. It goes something like this: The fastest way to get (pick one) heart disease, autism, glaucoma, vascular problems, osteoporosis, or any cancer is to be screened for it.

This book is about how to approach this tension.

Seeking Sickness raises the question of whether the so-called advances in diagnostic technology—our ability to see tiny anatomic abnormalities on scans and our ability to detect minute changes in our biochemical and genetic makeup—truly benefits those who are well.

Or does it simply lead to a lot of overdiagnosis and over-treatment?

It's a question worth thinking about.

After reading it you might reasonably conclude not to look to medical care to help make you healthy but instead to look to medical care to help you only if you get sick.

H. GILBERT WELCH, MD, MPH
Professor of Medicine
Dartmouth Institute for Health Policy & Clinical Practice

PROLOGUE

Seek and ye shall find

WE CAN find disease wherever we look; however, what do we lose in all the looking?

Medical screening is a powerful, seductive, and highly intuitive thing to do. After all, why wait until you have symptoms of a disease if you can take a simple test to help find it early? Especially early enough that you can do something about it?

These questions reverberate through one of the longest-running debates in health-care circles: the dichotomy of "prevention" versus "treatment."

Our health-care system by design ignores many of the factors that make us sick in the first place—which makes many people praise the logic of disease prevention in general and medical screening in particular. Proponents of this school use very compelling arguments, saying the billions we spend on disease prevention will save millions of lives, untold suffering, and countless billions on medical services down the road.

However, much of what passes for prevention—with medical screening as its centerpiece—is expensive, often misguided, and frequently counter-productive. Our collective efforts at seeking sickness often do nothing but promote health consumerism to the worried well, a phenomenon driven by private entrepreneurs, drug companies and medical specialists whose income depends on driving even more healthy people into screening.

Medical tests are extremely beneficial in discovering why you're sick, but what if you're healthy? That changes the equation mightily. It's this territory that this book sets out to examine.

Widespread screening of healthy people seems intuitively sound until you look a little closer and realize the costs and potential for harm are considerable. CT scanners are incredibly good at detecting tumors and arterial plaque, matched in these abilities by scientists who can find and then exploit markers in your genes, your organs, and your bones, which once uncovered, bring whole new problems to the fore, often without any benefits.

British physician Iona Heath, President of the Royal College of General Practitioners in the U.K., writes about the trend to put prevention above cure.[1] Governments around the world, influenced by many of the forces that profit from so-called preventive medicine, push the "screen early, screen often" rhetoric, driven by the "systematic exaggeration of the power of preventive medicine." As she puts it, "An excessive and unrealistic commitment to prevention of sickness could destroy our capacity to care for those who are already sick." Ultimately, prevention can only go so far, because "everyone, in time, must become sick and die."

A better understanding of why we are so energetically seeking sickness may raise more questions than it answers. But maybe that's what we need to have on hand—more questions, questions that help enforce a healthier "look before you leap" attitude—because when someone is coming at you with a medical screening test, those questions could be your parachute.

NOTE: Unless otherwise indicated, all $ amounts in this book refer to US$.

SEEKING SICKNESS

ONE

The whole body scan

Who's really reaping the benefits,
and why you don't need one

IF YOU live on an island like I do, you're never far away from water. My hometown is Victoria, British Columbia, and if I head out my front door and turn left, I have to walk for only ten minutes before I reach the shores of the Pacific Ocean. And at night when I'm down on the shore looking at the mountains, I can see the lights of a little seaside town of Port Angeles, Washington, twinkling across the 17 miles of water known as the Straits of Juan de Fuca. I get a certain comfort seeing that little town and its lights, nestled at the feet of those big snow-topped mountains. It reminds me how geographically and culturally Canadians and Americans are intertwined.

One morning a few years ago over breakfast, I was reading my local daily newspaper, the *Victoria Times Colonist,* when a yellow flyer fell out of the paper onto my lap. I was about to throw it in the recycling bin when the headline grabbed my eye:

"A full body scan can save your life."

In retrospect, this was a headline that ended up changing my life, but not in the way it was intended to.

To say I was intrigued is an understatement. Questions flooded over me: What the heck was this? Who was promising to save my life? How did they plan to save my life? And how much would they charge me to save my life? That's all? My life is worth $1,000? The more I thought about it, the more determined I was to get to the bottom of it.

The yellow flyer was an advertisement for a company that was operating a mobile screening unit doing scans in Port Angeles, Washington. The flyer was pitching high-tech screening of hearts, lungs, and arteries for a few hundred dollars each. And for the full enchilada—$1,000—a person could buy a full-body computed tomography (CT) scan, which, the headline claimed, could save your life.

A full-body scan typically focuses on three specific body areas—abdomen, lungs/chest, and brain—and it takes multiple pictures of each area to identify potential anomalies. It can also be done with a magnetic resonance imaging (MRI) machine. The full-body scan had been part of popular culture in the U.S. for more than five years when I saw that ad. In fact, in July 2002, the widely read magazine *Popular Mechanics* featured an article that captured the futuristic world of medical screening with references to *Star Trek*, saying that Dr. McCoy's examining room had moved "from the Starship *Enterprise* to your local mall."[1]

Sure to capture the unadulterated gee-whiz attention of more than just the Trekkies, this article said that "whole body medical scans will buy you peace of mind—or sleepless nights" and emphasized that "'Star Trek'-style whole-body scanning has become the hottest idea in medicine since computerized billing." Apparently, with tons of money to be made by offering full-body scans to healthy people, "doctors and investors are lining up to buy million-dollar-plus machines that painlessly turn your body inside out and look into your medical future." The rationale for doing such a scan was laid bare: "If your habits or your family history have put you at risk for developing cancer or heart disease, a whole-body scan could put your mind at ease."

Although the article was written almost like an advertisement for full-body screening, buried within it was this important caveat: "At the same time you get that clean bill of health, you may also discover a few things about your interior anatomy you would just as well have preferred not knowing."

I took the yellow flyer and showed it to my friends and colleagues, and more questions arose: Was this some kind of high-tech snake-oil scam? Can this stuff really save your life? If it was worthwhile, why wasn't our health system paying for it? If it wasn't worthwhile, was this marketing even legal? If it's a scam, who is protecting consumers from it? What if the scan finds something wrong with you? Who then pays for the surgeries and the biopsies and investigations that would follow? And could you get cancer from these new medical imaging tests?

It might have been my first experience of seeing companies like this pitching their wares—almost in the tones of a public service message—but then I started to see them everywhere. And I also saw the homegrown versions in the bigger Canadian cities; private companies that were trying to muscle in on medical screening, offering peace of mind with the promise of a full-body scan.

This was unusual. Canadians are often described as "Americans with public health care," so in our collective minds there is something about opening our wallets for medical services that bothers us. Many have come to believe if a medical procedure is necessary and important, then the government will pay for it. If the government doesn't, the procedure might be neither necessary nor important.

But this? This full body–scanning thing?

I did what any self-respecting researcher does when an idea in need of investigation strikes: I tried to find out what the research literature said on full-body scanning. It was sparse; so with a few colleagues, I wrote a grant proposal to get some funds to look deeper. I wanted to methodically sift through the evidence, interview the experts both in Canada and abroad, and examine the regulations. I also wanted to make sure we had enough money to do some polling.

My thinking was this: It's of huge importance to discover what the public thinks of the value of full-body scans and other screening technologies. I also wanted to know if people were as shocked as I was that an American company was offering to save our lives for $1,000.

Within the federal department of Industry Canada (whose job is to flog the products of Canada's industries) is a tiny branch called the Office of Consumer Affairs. That branch gives annual grants to fund consumer-oriented research. Consumer Affairs must have liked our pitch, because within four months we had a nonprofit partner and some money to study and publish our results.[2]

Suffice to say, things were worse than I'd expected.

Like our brethren south of the border, Canadians were being exposed to the marketing by private companies of health-screening services such as heart, lung, and full-body scans using CT (computed tomography) or PET (positron emission tomography) within our own borders. We also found that these clinics were owned and/or operated by businessman radiologists who also provide services to provincial medicare plans and work in hospitals. And there was overwhelming evidence that CT, MRI, PET, or CT/PET scans were not accurate enough to warrant their use in whole-body screening of healthy populations. We found these services weren't benign and that full-body scans carry the risk of misdiagnosis, overdiagnosis, and unnecessary subsequent testing.

One of the more shocking findings was that submitting to a full-body screen usually led to a whole lot more screening. In one study of 1,192 patients (76 percent of whom were self-referred) who got whole-body CT scans at a community screening center, 86 percent of them were told they had an abnormal finding. Of those, more than one-third (37 percent) were referred for follow-up examinations, which meant more imaging.[3]

Scans can be expensive but not as expensive or invasive as all the follow-up investigations, tests, scans, surgeries, biopsies, and hospital care that would happen if anything unusual were found. The problem is that most of the "unusual" things found by full-body scanning are benign and not significant in the absence of symptoms or other clinical history.

If full-body scanning took off, all the follow-up performed on benign anomalies could wreak havoc on any medical system. And one of the biggest issues for any government in Canada is whether we can keep public health care sustainable to treat an aging population. More full-body screening would mean a lot more health care and a lot more money. The $1,000 for the test was just the beginning.

"The test is chump change. It's all the stuff that happens afterward that costs a lot," says Dr. H. Gilbert Welch, the author of *Overdiagnosed: Making People Sick in Pursuit of Health* (written with Drs. Steven Woloshin and Lisa Schwartz). This is not a tiny problem in Welch's estimation. In fact, he says the whole system of detecting medical abnormalities that will never go on to harm you is the "the biggest problem posed by modern medicine."

In addition to the follow-up and medical investigations that might result from a false positive, the radiation a person is exposed to in the course of a scan must be considered. The radiation exposure from full-body CT scans could vary a lot, by as much as 35 percent, depending on the machine used, the settings, the operator, and so on. Health Canada's website says that a single chest CT scan delivers radiation equal to between 500 and 1,000 chest X-rays. A report in the U.K.[4] said that "the radiation exposure from a whole body CT scan is between 4 and 24 mSv (biologically effective dose). An effective dose of 10 mSv (equivalent to 500 chest radiographs) results in a risk of cancer death of 1 in 2,000." In the U.S., it is estimated that 1.5 percent to 2 percent of cancers at present can be attributed to radiation exposure from CT scanning. The exposure also varies depending on the settings used because of the way full-body CT scans are done: the proto-cols that the clinics or hospitals use are not standardized.[5]

Other countries have different rules. In some countries (for example, Germany and Switzerland), the use of any screening test that involves radiation exposure is forbidden by law.[6]

Then there is the problem of operator error. The findings of a CT scan depend on who is interpreting the scan. One study found a 37 percent disagreement rate between radiologists' interpreta-tions of the results of a CT body scan. Another found a 32 percent discrepancy rate between initial interpretation and reinterpreta-tions of abdominal CT scans.[7]

Some people might ask, well, why don't I just get a full-body MRI, which doesn't use radiation? It's a good question, but also not without its issues. Although MRI scans do not carry the risk of ionizing radiation, they can (when used to screen healthy people) detect abnormalities that may never have been a problem, lead-ing to unnecessary treatment and cost.[8] An MRI also exposes the body to a different kind of powerful energy field that can torque a metal implant in the body, and repeated exposure may ultimately be found to cause problems. Having an MRI scan may also entail use of a contrast dye that can harm some people.

But is there any real benefit to be had from full-body screen-ing? A 2006 study found that providing full-body CT screening to a group of 500,000 healthy people at age 50 would lead to an average gain in life expectancy of only 6 days in 26.3 years. The same study estimates that false-positive results accounted for about 30 percent of the total costs.[9]

Our little research study couldn't find anyone—neither sci-entists nor the scientific literature, nor professional or regulatory bodies—who agreed with the "save your life" claims made by the companies promoting full-body scans. The executives of the com-panies waffled when we interviewed them, aware that they didn't have any quality research to back up their claims. But that didn't stop them from marketing their services from a dozen different centers in Canada and hundreds in the U.S.

Incredibly, we discovered that using high-tech cancer-scanning technologies on asymptomatic people (specifically heart, lung, and full-body scans) was like riding into the Wild West, where anything goes. The medical screening entrepreneurs were pounding them back in the Free Enterprise Saloon, and the poor citizens of Dodge had no sheriff to protect them.

It would be a stretch to say that full-body scans were being regulated at all—at least regulated in any way that the unsuspecting consumer would construe as "consumer protection." We found that even the U.S. Food and Drug Administration (FDA) did not regulate how clinics use CT scans, and the only relevant comments they seemed to have were on the effectiveness of them. They said that they "know of no scientific evidence demonstrating that whole-body scanning of individuals without symptoms provides more benefit than harm to people being screened."[10]

But are consumers being protected? This is a gray area. The FDA oversees the effectiveness and safety of medical devices, and it says it "prohibits manufacturers of CT systems to promote their use for whole-body screening of asymptomatic people." Really? What about all those billboards, Internet ads, and flyers that plop out of newspapers? There's a caveat there: The FDA "does not regulate practitioners and they may choose to use a device for any use they deem appropriate."[11]

It seems that regulators around the world are having trouble regulating how CT scanning is promoted to the general public by private entrepreneurs. Even as the FDA prohibits manufacturers of CT systems from promoting them to healthy people as full-body scan technology, the practitioners seem to be flogging them for whatever kind of screening the market will bear. And in the U.K., two senior medical officials wrote to the Health Secretary to complain that "some private companies are taking advantage of vulnerable people by claiming that the health screening they offer will detect diseases early or reduce an individual's risk of developing specific illnesses." Dr. Hamish Meldrum, British Medical Association council chairman, said that even though the National

Health Service has safeguards in place to protect the public, "such safeguards often do not exist in the private sector, which makes it impossible for people to distinguish between private testing services that may do some good, and those that are of no value or even potentially harmful."[12]

Unlike the way the pharmaceutical industry is regulated in countries like Canada, the U.S., and Australia, where products are tested in extensive trials, approved by the regulator, and then monitored when they are on the market, there were no such restrictions on anyone who wanted to set up a private screening lab in Canada (or draw Canadians to the U.S. where they could get such tests). Both the regulation of practitioners and private clinics falls under the jurisdiction of provinces (and of states in the U.S.) and self-regulatory professional bodies.

But what was the average Joe in the streets thinking about all this? We finished this project by carrying out a Canada-wide public opinion survey of 400 Canadians on perceptions of this type of screening.

I wanted to do the survey for one simple reason: If there were Canadians being exposed to this kind of marketing for private screening, what did they think about it? Did they want it? Did they want to pay for it? And did they think it was safe?

Our poll results revealed that consumers are wildly misinformed about the reliability of different screening tests, and that there are very few sources of consumer-oriented, high-quality information about the use of these medical imaging procedures for screening. We found that 65 percent of respondents indicated that they believed that the detection of a potential health problem with a private CT scan would contribute to a longer life. Nearly half the people surveyed indicated that CT scans can verify the absence of disease at least 80 percent of the time.

Consumers also had grossly mistaken expectations regarding safety and regulatory oversight concerning these tests, erroneously believing that Canadian governments actively regulated the different uses and advertising of medical imaging screening tests provided through private imaging clinics.

The findings of our survey were not entirely unexpected. Prior to conducting it, I had, as a reality check, showed the yellow flyer to two American physicians who I was sure could provide insight into the kind of messages such advertising is sending to consumers. Drs. Steven Woloshin and Lisa M. Schwartz are long-time physician researchers and educators who are keenly interested in raising the bar on health literacy in the U.S. They are co-authors with Dr. H. Gilbert Welch of the book *Know Your Chances: Understanding Health Statistics*. All three are practicing physicians at the Veterans Administration Medical Center in White River Junction, Vermont. Their work with physicians, consumers, and journalists over the years has focused on helping people make sense of the whirling vortex of medical statistics. They have seen their share of drug and other health-care advertising that bombards consumers and paints dire risks to our health, then offers lifesaving solutions.

Dr. Woloshin jumped in first. "It's pretty outrageous. I mean, 'A body scan can save your life?'" he intoned quizzically. He flipped it over to look at the other side: "This is the ad that lets consumers choose amongst a bunch of scans."[13]

He then read the ad's pitch: "'Experts say most heart disease, strokes, and cancer can be prevented by being discovered early'?"

"It's a crazy ad," he said, "because the screening can find these things but they can't prevent them. You're not preventing anything. Maybe they meant the scan can prevent death from them." He sounded a little irritated as he blurted out, "Then the ad is just a lie. Because there is no credible evidence that these scans prevent death from anything." He mentioned that there might be some small exceptions in selected people but added, "there's lots of reasons to think they may do more harm than good."

Dr. Schwartz eagerly chimed in: "In fact, the thyroid included in the full-body scan is a test where people who are training to do scans are actually told *do not look at the thyroid gland*, because there are so many abnormalities in the thyroid gland. We know that most of those abnormalities should not be found. Actually, you'll be harming people by finding them." She looks over the list of different organ screenings offered and said, "In fact, some of these tests are clearly harmful."

She'd seen a lot of this kind of advertising—the marketing of fear to get people to submit to these tests. And she recalled an older message she'd heard from the American Cancer Society when it was running a campaign promoting mammograms.

"Their message was: '*Women who don't get a mammogram need more than their breasts examined,*'" she said. "So here it's only an insane woman who would forgo mammography? Telling people there's no choice?"

I wondered why the American Cancer Society would resort to such a condescending message. Schwartz surmised that when you've got a test you think is lifesaving, you need to pull out the stops to convince people to take it.

"There's a sense 'by any means necessary'—we have to get people to do this test." She said, "There's lots of psychological theories to get people to do something. There is a need to emotionally engage them, shock them sometimes, with fear."

But, I wondered, who is driving this fearmongering?

As Woloshin said, "Sometimes with pharmaceutical-company ads or industry-based ads, someone will clearly benefit—the manufacturer of the resource." But, he added, referring to screening or groups that are out there promoting flu shots, "with these public health announcements, it's less clear who directly benefits. Sometimes it's the true believer and the person involved in that aspect of public health. They need to try to convince everyone." Nonetheless, he said, "instead of helping people make an informed decision, for whatever reason they use these persuasive messages to get people to do what they think is right for them."

And apparently some of that convincing works. Schwartz and Woloshin conducted a study back in 2004[14] to see whether these kinds of consumer-targeted health ads were working. They did some public opinion survey work around the time that the marketing of full-body scans was at its height in the U.S.

Schwartz explained her work: "Why we wanted to do this study is to understand the effect of these public health messages and how this creates an environment that is ripe for the dissemination of a message that says 'Earlier is better.'" The messages reinforced the common ideology behind screening, "that you're a good person if you start looking for disease earlier."

Schwartz and Woloshin conducted a phone poll of 500 adults from across the U.S.—men and women for whom cancer tests were recommended. Through their data, a very clear picture came into focus. Schwartz said, "Americans are incredibly enthusiastic about cancer screening—they thought it was almost *always* a good idea. So much so that they would overrule a physician who recommended that they not get a screening."

The stats that emerged from Schwartz and Woloshin's survey were somewhat surprising: 74 percent of those surveyed believed that finding cancer early would save a person's life "most or all the time."

"In fact, it goes further than this," said Schwartz. "Few could imagine a time when they would stop getting screened. In fact, this enthusiasm was not damped by having a false positive."

This floored me. After all, I thought, once bitten, twice shy, right? Wouldn't someone who lives through a cancer scare resulting from a screen like a mammogram or a PSA test lose enthusiasm for subsequent screening? Don't people really hate it when others cry wolf?

"Not at all," said Schwartz, referring to people who had false positives. "Even though they said it was scary and some said it was the scariest time of their life, almost all of them were glad they had the test. Because in the end, [with] the reassurance of finding out that they didn't have cancer, they didn't see the false positive as a harmful experience but a reassuring experience."

That changed my mind about what people think of screening. But it also reinforced a theme that you will find throughout this book. When people are screened, and the screening "finds something," and they are treated, they typically believe a single thing: that their lives have been saved. And then they go on to become foot soldiers and activists in the war on breast cancer, prostate cancer, and so on.

But when you look into what the average American thinks about high-tech screening you see how money influences a person's thoughts about health care. For example, researchers in one study found that people getting a CT scan felt they were getting better health care than if they didn't get one.

One study surveyed people reporting to the ER with non-traumatic abdominal pain and concluded that "patients are more confident when CT imaging is part of their medical evaluation but have a poor understanding of the concomitant radiation exposure and risk and underestimate their previous imaging experience."[15]

What this leads to is probably many more people are getting scans they don't need. Again, it's worth reminding ourselves that we're talking about screening: doing scans on well people and trying to find things wrong with them. When a person who has symptoms gets a scan so that his or her doctor can diagnose what's wrong, that scan is a *diagnostic test*—not screening. The extent to which people are getting unnecessary scans is hard to quantify, but recent research on this issue estimated that approximately one-third of all CT scans in the U.S. are "not justified by medical need."[16]

So what was driving all the screening, other than the profound belief that it must be good for all of us, all of the time? Clearly there was a demand, even though we found that in Canada, full-body CT scans could cost upwards of $1,000,[17] were not recommended by independent experts or professional bodies, had no quality data supporting their benefits, and were capable of delivering doses of radiation that statistically caused a small number of people to actually develop cancer somewhere down the road. What was happening here? Was it the force of marketing or the seductive lure of "doing something" to prevent disease? Or was it the "Oprah effect"?

Woloshin and Schwartz surveyed Americans with a question that we replicated with Canadians several years later. "Which would you rather have: a full-body CT scan or $1,000?" The majority of the Americans, more than 70 percent in Woloshin and Schwartz's study,[18] as well as about 63 percent of Canadians in my survey,[19] said they'd rather have the full-body scan, expressing what I thought was a surprising enthusiasm (and ignorance) of this new, unproven, and probably dangerous test. But you can't discount the power of a celebrity endorsement.

Lisa qualified her results by saying, "We did this survey at the peak time of enthusiasm in the U.S. Oprah underwent a full-body CT. She told the story on the show. It followed a story in USA *Today.* And so on…"

Like many things that experience the joys of the Oprah effect, full-body scanning has had a boost because of it. And in 2006, Oprah had a CT scan of her heart to detect cardiovascular disease, and she urged other women to do the same, saying, "Don't be one of those crazy people who doesn't want the information."[20]

Schwartz tells me that originally her survey hadn't set out to ask about the full-body scan, and that they were talking to people about several proven screening tests. As they were surveying people, several respondents said, "I want that test that Oprah was talking about."

One big problem with getting a scan is the rate of "inappropriate reassurance." The screener tells you that you are disease free when, in fact, you're anything but. This situation is also called the false-negative phenomenon. A 2007 report in the U.K. looking at the impact of healthy-person scanning with CT said the following:

A negative scan—even a true negative scan—may lead to a belief by the individual that they are "healthy"; this idea is certainly implied by the advertising of many private companies operating in this area. There is a wide range of life-limiting conditions, however, which are not addressed by asymptomatic whole-body CT scanning, e.g., obesity, hypertension, hyperlipidemia, diabetes and some forms of cancer.[21]

The idea is that if people are told that they're normal, they might carry on with an unhealthy lifestyle in the belief that they've got a perfect bill of health.

Who else is benefiting from pushing full-body screening?

Clearly the physicians who work in the screening field benefit from it, and they may be prone to seeing only the benefits and not the harms of their work. Most professionals involved in whole-body screening would have a strong belief in the value of the service they offer (hence the need for independent information and regulators).

As far back as ten years ago, physicians with the American College of Radiology (the professional body governing radiologists in the U.S.) and the Canadian Association of Radiologists (its counterpart in Canada) were expressing skepticism around pushing whole-body scanning on a naïve and ignorant public. Their concerns around whole-body scans might have been best summed up by Dr. Harald Stolberg of McMaster University, who questioned the utility, ethics, and cost-effectiveness of the scans, saying, "The only known benefit of this marketing ploy is the financial advantage to the radiologists or the organizations providing CT screening."[22]

The momentum of the full-body scan industry has slowed in the last several years due to criticism from professional organizations.[23] Some companies may still try to flog full-body scans to the unsuspecting public, but there is a sense that, as with *Star Trek*, there is only nostalgia left for the era of the "full-body scam."

Lisa Schwartz says that she is "puzzled by the decline of the full-body scan—although it's not extinct." She has a few theories, including the idea that the popular press is getting the word out that the radiation doses are high. In response to the growing public awareness of the potential radiation hazards of CT-screening, scanning companies are promoting other methods—such as full-body MRI scans—on the basis of their safety.

She says, "The idea of scanning in other forms with ultra-sounds via for-profit companies in the U.S., like Lifeline, is still very popular. So it's possible that just the mechanism of scanning is changing rather than the attitude."

Dr. Nortin M. Hadler, a U.S. physician and author of several popular books, including *Worried Sick: A Prescription for Health in an Overtreated America* and *The Last Well Person: How to Stay Well Despite the Health-Care System,* has an excellent reputation for debunking consumer-oriented medical myths. Dr. Hadler has a different theory on why full-body screening might be a dying market in North America: "I think it reflects the fact that it's an out-of-pocket expense, and most pockets are empty."[24]

The march of the full-body scan might be slowing in both Canada and the U.S., but as I go down to the beach in my hometown to watch the ships sailing past heading to Asia, something inside me says that at least some of those container ships heading east to China or India are probably carrying screening technology. At the very least, North America is exporting its ideology of "screen early and screen often," which may find a much more receptive audience in those developing economies whose citizens want to buy the things that middle-class people elsewhere buy—including $1,000 high-tech full-body scans.

The business press supports my suspicions. A recent report by PricewaterhouseCoopers[25] said that American companies dominate the $350 billion–per-year global medical device industry, and in these times of economic doom and gloom, the medical device industry is one of the few sectors that show a positive trade balance.

TWO

Screening for eyeball pressure

Know the right questions to ask (for any screening test) and when to ask them

BECAUSE OF my research into screening technology, I thought that I was probably better armed than most people against its frivolous use. But self-delusion can sometimes be so, well, self-deluding.

I didn't see myself as someone easily pushed in the direction of unnecessary medical screening, but it wasn't until I was sitting in the optometrist's chair that I realized an embarrassing truth: I was absolutely horrible at practicing what I preached.

Since I'd begun researching medical screening, I'd always said (to anyone who asked) that the main thing you need to do to protect yourself from the adverse effects of medical screening was your research. Then you needed to ask a few key, possibly lifesaving questions.

By the time I was at the optometrist's, I'd been researching and writing about medical screening for over a year. I'd interviewed experts and trolled through guidelines created by such august bodies as the World Health Organization (WHO) and the U.S. Preventive Services Task Force (USPSTF). I had talked to patients who were helped by screening as well as those who'd had their lives turned upside down by it. I was wary but had taken many lessons to heart. I was slowly concluding that to make an informed decision about whether to be screened, people needed to be armed with good questions on the overall benefits and harms of screening.

Which is to say, us ordinary folk need to be much more suspicious of the "do this test because it will be good for you" mantra that screening marketers and practitioners often chant to us.

So imagine this scene. My wife suggested that it was time for me to get my eyes tested. Of course, I bristled. My glasses were fine, and I had no problem seeing. Besides, hadn't I just had my eyes examined? But that was a year and a half ago.

So I plunked down $105 at an optometry clinic to get an eye exam. The exam itself was the standard optometrist stuff, with me being asked if I could see (or not see) the various rows of letters flashed up on the wall. The optometrist could tell right away whether my eyesight had deteriorated since the last visit and how much my eyeglass prescription had changed.

But then he pulled out a tool that my Spidey senses told me was part of some kind of screening test. If I'd been wearing a blood-pressure cuff at the time, I'm sure you'd have been able to measure my reaction in the climbing numbers.

Could it be true, I asked myself, that I was about to face the pointy end of an actual screening test?

That's exactly what was happening.

I tried to remain calm. After all, what could be wrong with having an optometrist puff a bit of air into your eye to see if you've got "high eyeball pressure?" The optometrist pulled out the little tool, which I later learned is called a noncontact tonometer. It was about the size of a telephone handset and is used to measure intraocular pressure (IOP).

I wanted to know what he was going to do with the thing. Our conversation went something like this:

Alan: What's that for? Are you doing a screening test on me?

Optometrist: Yes, it's a screening test. Just a little puff of air against your cornea. It measures the pressure of the fluid cycling inside the eye.

Alan: [*clearly interested*] So why do you need to know the pressure inside my eyeball?

Optometrist: It's just a little test that can tell us whether the fluid in your eyeball pressure is normal. High pressure might lead to glaucoma.

Alan: What's that?

Optometrist: Glaucoma is a condition in which the optic nerve gets damaged. It affects your vision. This test can show if you've got high intraocular pressure, which might lead to some risk of developing glaucoma. Glaucoma can lead to blindness.

Alan: [*getting a little testy*] Are you telling me that you're about to test my eyes with a puff of air, and that puffer you're holding will tell you I've got a chance of being blind in the future?

Optometrist: Not really. It's just a quick screen of your pressure. If the reading is high, I'd talk to you about what it could potentially mean, and there's a few other diagnostic tests we would do. There could be a number of things causing the pressure in your eyeball to rise, so we'd do more tests to rule out those things. We'd also check out the visual field. If glaucoma damage is happening, you're going to find it symptomatically in the visual field.

Alan: So this is just the first slice, right? This screening test?

Optometrist: Yes. By the way, why are you asking so many questions?

Alan: I've been researching a lot about screening lately. In fact, I'm writing a book about it. You know, I've always wondered why when facing a screening test (like I am right now), people don't ask the right questions. This feels weird. It's actually hard to think of the right questions when you're on the spot like this.

Optometrist: [*reassuringly*] Yeah, it's a pretty simple test, but it's not definitive and it won't lead to anything. We'd have to do a whole bunch of other diagnostic tests if we thought something was wrong.

If it was obvious to him that I was stalling for time, he didn't show it. But I was running out of questions. I was flummoxed and gave in. What happened next took about five seconds. He puffed a shot of air into each of my eyeballs and said, "Your pressure is normal—it's 21," and then carried on with the rest of my eye exam.

This was a moment of strong self-realization. Now I had the inside scoop on what it felt like to be asked to take a screening test. But if I'd given it more thought, I would have realized that the whole visit to the optometrist is a screening test. I'm perfectly healthy and handing myself over to get checked for disease.

Much of my writing exhorted people to take all the time they need to do their research and ask questions before being screened. But things look different when you're sitting in the chair, playing the role of the trusting patient. It was like I had two angels sitting on my shoulders. One was whispering in one ear: "What's the big deal? It was just a puff of air to the eyes. C'mon." On the other shoulder, the naysayer angel, armed with a pitchfork, was jabbing me in the ear: "Are you nuts? Do you have any idea what this screening test will lead to? False positives. False negatives. Overdiagnosis. Downstream effects. Worry. Anxiety. Depression. Say no!"

OK, I'm being overdramatic. The lesson here seemed pretty simple: If you are about to face a health professional who might offer you a screening test, you need to have already done your research. Doing it afterward is getting things backward.

The research on how people make decisions related to screening is not very robust—which is a nice way to say that there isn't much of it that's of any use. Yet the "Decisions Study" in 2010 in the United States surveyed citizens nationwide asking about nine common medical decisions and how informed patients felt they were about those decisions.[1]

The study concluded that "cancer screening discussions across all screening tests (breast, colorectal, prostate)" rated poorly in terms of "criteria for informed decision making." Which tells me people weren't getting the information they needed to make an informed decision. Either they didn't ask for it or it wasn't provided.

The study went on to say that "participants reported that health care providers frequently failed to discuss the cons of screening and did not routinely elicit patient preferences." Even if people thought they were well informed, "they performed poorly in answering knowledge questions and significantly overestimated incidence and mortality risks and the predictive values of PSA tests and mammography."

What this says to me is that even before you get offered a screening test, you should be doing your homework (unlike me *not* doing my homework before visiting the optometrist).

Later, when I did my research, I discovered that it is recommended that we periodically have our eyes examined for a simple reason: many of the diseases of our eyes don't have any symptoms. In other words, we don't feel any differently even if there is something wrong with us.

Some eye examinations are able to detect things that could lead to blindness (such as early signs of high eyeball pressure that could lead to glaucoma). And sometimes, diseases that have nothing to do with our eyes (such as diseases of the brain) can be detected in anomalies in our eyes.

There are a number of ways to measure eyeball pressure. The noncontact tonometry (or air-puff tonometry) my optometrist used on me employs a shot of air to flatten the cornea. The machine turns this into a reading that translates into IOP. High pressure can be treated with eyedrops.

But back to why I agreed to this screening test.

For starters, imminent blindness is a pretty strong motivator. Losing your eyesight would be a pretty traumatic thing, and if a health professional is offering a screening tool that can detect the early signs of it, and the test seems simple and noninvasive, with few downstream risks, why wouldn't you go ahead with it? Isn't this the rationale around any screening test? But I knew there was more to it. With any screening test, there is always some profit motive lurking in the background. There is therefore a strong financial incentive for that screening to be used as frequently and as widely as possible.

For companies that make and sell pressure-lowering eyedrops, is there an incentive to exaggerate the need for eyeball screening? They are certainly motivated to promote the link between lowering your eye pressure with drugs and a reduction in the potential for glaucoma. The drug maker Pfizer, for instance, has a campaign called "All Eyes on Glaucoma" that recommends regular glaucoma screening, including tonometry.[2] They also sell the widely marketed drug latanoprost (or Xalatan)—eyedrops designed to reduce eyeball pressure. The makers of handheld tonometers would also benefit from exaggerating the role that increased eye pressure plays in glaucoma.

Yet the deeper I dug into eyeball-pressure screening, the more I discovered that the jury was still out on it. One study, the "Ocular Hypertension Treatment Study,"[3] found that screening for ocular hypertension and treating people for it meant that those people were less likely to develop glaucoma compared to a control group. But there's a catch. High eyeball pressure is only a risk factor for glaucoma. Most people with high eyeball pressure do not develop glaucoma. In fact 25 percent to 50 percent of people with glaucoma have normal eye pressure.

There is also uncertainty over the accuracy of tonometry because eyeball pressure changes throughout the day. In addition, the test does not account for differences in thickness and curvature of the cornea from patient to patient, and some methods rely a great deal on the operator. Yet some manufacturers are even selling a handheld home tonometry device so that you can check your own eyeball pressure as often as you like.

Many organizations, such as the Glaucoma Foundation in the U.S. and the Canadian National Institute for the Blind, recommend routine eye-pressure checks but are possibly misleading people about how well the test can detect glaucoma. From what I've found, the benefit of routine eye-pressure testing is probably exaggerated beyond the evidence, and there are simply not enough quality studies looking specifically at the long-term results of tonometry screening. But that doesn't mean you should avoid getting a routine eye test. After all, it's not like they're going to cut out part of your lung on the basis of a false positive.

I admit my timing was off: I did all this research *after* I'd undergone the eye-pressure screening test. Prior to my experience in the optometrist's chair, I had always wondered why people didn't ask more questions when confronted with a screening test. Now I knew. You never know when someone medical is going to offer you a screening test. And it's hard to say no when you're there, already sitting in the chair.

Therefore expect to be screened and be prepared, armed with a few good questions.

Since then, I've developed a list of six questions one needs to ask when being offered a screening test:

1. *Is this screening test recommended by a quality independent body, such as the U.S. Preventive Services Task Force (USPSTF)?*
2. *Is it for a disease that significantly impacts public health, is prevalent enough to require screening, and comes with an acceptable probability that I could have it?*
3. *If my doctor detects pre-disease, will it be at a point at which a cure can be enacted for the disease that could follow?*
4. *Is the test sensitive (meaning it can accurately find disease that IS there), and is it specific (meaning that it won't find disease that ISN'T there)?*
5. *Who is pushing this test, and why?*
6. *If I have a positive test, what does further evaluation look like, and is medical care available to effectively treat this disease in a manner that I find acceptable?*

And always, regardless of the test offered, determine first that it is safe and well tolerated by those it is performed upon.

I'll answer each of the questions below in the context of an eyeball-pressure test, but they can be used for any type of screening.

1. *Is this screening test recommended by a quality, independent body such as the USPSTF?*

"The USPSTF found good evidence that screening can detect increased intraocular pressure (IOP) and early primary open-angle glaucoma (POAG) in adults. The USPSTF also found good evidence that early treatment of adults with increased IOP detected by screening reduces the number of persons who develop small visual-field defects, and that early treatment of those with early, asymptomatic POAG decreases the number of those whose visual-field defects progress."[4]

But here's the kicker: "The evidence, however, is insufficient to determine the extent to which screening—leading to the earlier detection and treatment of people with IOP or POAG—would reduce impairment in vision-related function or quality of life." The Canadian Agency for Drugs and Technologies in Health summarized the various guidelines regarding tonometry and found that there isn't a consensus on the benefits of eye-pressure screening or one on who should be screened.[5]

Translation: The jury is still out. Maybe earlier detection can lead to reducing vision-related problems in the future. Or maybe it won't.

2. *Is it for a disease that significantly impacts public health, is prevalent enough to require screening, and comes with an acceptable probability that I could have it?*

According to the World Glaucoma Association, glaucoma is the second most common cause of blindness worldwide. It is estimated that 4.5 million persons globally are blind due to glaucoma. About 7 percent of all patients with glaucoma are younger than 55 years of age, 44 percent are between 55 and 74 years, and

49 percent are older than 74 years.[6] The number-one risk factor is age. My optometrist also said this, so that was reassuring, as I was 47 at the time of the test. However, being screened for a condition still exposes me to the risks of false positives and false negatives.

3. *If my doctor detects pre-disease, will it be at a point at which a cure can be enacted for the disease that could follow?*

In the case of the eyeball-pressure test, if I'd had a high result, other diagnostic tests would have been done to see if there was damage to my optic nerve. There are also prescription drugs available to treat high eyeball pressure, usually eyedrops. One randomized trial concluded that "topical ocular hypotensive medication was effective in delaying or preventing the onset of Primary Open-Angle Glaucoma (POAG) in individuals with elevated IOP." It does, however, go on to say that "this does not imply that all patients with borderline or elevated IOP should receive medication."[7] In my case, a "normal" reading does not necessarily mean an automatic clean bill of health.

4. *Is the test sensitive (meaning it can accurately find disease that IS there), and is it specific (meaning that it won't find disease that ISN'T there)?*

The authors of a 2001 paper advocate for glaucoma screening and stress that several methods of detection should be used. "With the use of a single device such as tonometry, the probability of a false-positive glaucoma diagnosis is high." One report on a glaucoma-screening program in the U.S. (the Student Sight Savers Program) found that the method of noncontact tonometry employed by the program had a sensitivity of only 22.1 percent and a specificity of 78.6 percent.[8] Remember, sensitivity is reflected by the percentage of screened people who have the condition and are correctly identified as such. It is also called the true positive rate. If one in five is correctly identified as having high eyeball pressure, that certainly leaves a lot of room for other explanations. Specificity refers to the percentage of screened people who don't have the condition being accurately identified by the test as not having it. It is also called the true negative rate. In this case, four out of five people who don't have the condition are correctly identified as such, and that sounds pretty good.

We should remember that no test has a 100 percent sensitivity and 100 percent specificity. Therefore, we must be prepared to look for other clues to discover if there is true sickness there or true health. Both conditions shuold be identified properly.

According to some critics of this kind of screening, the gold-standard test for intraocular pressure depends too much on the operator.[9] Some say the tonometer does not take into account the differences in corneal curvature and thickness from patient to patient.[10] As one researcher said, "Tonometry is a poor screening tool because a large proportion of patients with glaucoma don't have elevated IOP—and, conversely, a large proportion of people have high IOP but no glaucoma."[11]

5. *Who is pushing this test, and why?*

Optometrists, drug companies who make eyedrops and other glaucoma treatments, as well as makers of tonometers promote glaucoma screening. One company, for example, promotes World Glaucoma Day by offering free screening events. No doubt those events not only help highlight the importance of eyeball screening but also help showcase and promote that company's products.[12] Is there anything wrong with these activities? No. But information provided by those with financial interests in screening must be consumed in the knowledge that it's probably biased.

6. *If I have a positive test, what does further evaluation look like, and is medical care available to effectively treat this disease in a manner that I find acceptable?*

Not everyone who has higher than normal eyeball pressure needs to be treated with drugs to lower the pressure. The eyedrops used to lower intraocular pressure can cause changes in eye color, stinging, blurred vision, redness, itching, and burning. Some decrease blood pressure or may cause memory problems and kidney stones.[13]

And is this test safe and well tolerated? Tonometer tips for certain types of tonometers can be a source of hepatitis and other infections if they are not properly disinfected.[14] And is the test well tolerated? Most people find the test only slightly uncomfortable.

At the end of the day, I was glad I had the tonometry exam as it was a good test flight into the screening world. The whole experience gave me some insight into how crucial it is to do one's research beforehand and be ready with questions. It's important to know why a screening test is being offered and what could happen if it shows something abnormal. I am not currently living under a cloud of fear that I may have glaucoma brewing in my eyes, but what if my pressure had been "high"? Would my mental state be different now? Would I be worried that I could one day go blind? Would this worry affect how I live the rest of my life? And furthermore, even though I had a normal result, have the seeds of doubt been planted in my head?

If you have gotten this far in my book it's because you have some interest in screening. Here's a suggestion: Keep the above questions in mind as you read the upcoming chapters, which present some of the research on the most commonly used screening tests.

And if you can't remember all the questions when you face a real-life screening test, try remembering just this one: "Doctor, what happens if I do nothing?"

THREE

Cholesterol screening, syndrome X, and heart scanning

The risky business of screening for risk

ANY DISEASE that represents the number-one cause of death globally is going to be a big target for disease prevention and medical screening. According to the World Health Organization (WHO), cardiovascular disease—illness affecting the heart or blood vessels—is a serious killer, representing 30 percent of all deaths worldwide. While most medical advice might focus on a healthier lifestyle as a preventive—eating better, not smoking, exercising, and so on—doctors often screen for signs of disease in our blood, blood vessels, and sometimes our hearts. When they clamp a blood pressure cuff on you, or send you to the lab for a cholesterol test, they are, in effect, screening you for disease. Although it might seem innocuous to be screening for risk factors (such as high cholesterol) or clusters of risk factors (as is the case with "syndrome X"), there is always the potential for this screening to end badly.

George Thompson (not his real name) from Richmond, British Columbia, is a dutiful patient who follows his doctor's advice.

Among other things, he gets an annual blood test to monitor his various blood measurements, primarily blood sugar and cholesterol. Even though he likes to tell the doctor that there's no heart disease in his family and that most of his ancestors lived until they were old, he went along with the tests anyway. It's what one does.

Yet, those drops of blood taken from his vein to be screened by medical professionals in a trusted and reliable way would change his life forever.

At age 51, George's routine blood test indicated that he had high cholesterol. His doctor told him he needed to modify his diet and start taking Lipitor, a medication from the drug group called statins. Later, his doctor moved him to another drug, Crestor, also a statin. In addition, he was also taking two drugs for his high blood pressure.

Initially, George was happy with his doctor's advice about the high cholesterol. "My doctor just walked me through the numbers and explained what it all meant."[1]

He was taking Lipitor and then Crestor, and it wasn't until seven years later that "all the shit happened." He said it was "one thing after another. It included sharp pain to my lower abdomen that got occasionally so sharp that it took my breath away."

The worst part for him was the noticeable muscle wasting he saw in his shoulders, which used to be broad but after years on cholesterol drugs started to look withered. "I was starting to look like a snake, with no shoulders," he recalls.

Finally, George had had enough of the muscle weakening and the other symptoms, so he stopped taking all his drugs. Cold turkey.

"I didn't know what was doing me harm. So I quit them all. I'd had enough of all this B.S."

Perhaps it was George's intuition, but it's not unreasonable for people who have no previous heart disease to wonder why they need to take a statin drug to lower their cholesterol. In fact, some might say that cholesterol screening is a routine medical practice that needs a serious rethink.

Dr. Nortin M. Hadler has written a number of popular books helping people draw the line between rational health care and medical marketing. He tackles the question of screening for and treating high cholesterol in his latest book, *Rethinking Aging: Growing Old and Living Well in an Overtreated Society.* He calls much of such testing a "risk factor fetish."[2]

Perhaps Dr. Hadler's books are so popular because his recommendations come from a solid medical background and even more solid common sense. He writes that he refuses to have his own blood checked for high cholesterol.

In his words, "cholesterol is a weak risk factor in well people, but there is also no compelling evidence that even if my cholesterol was 'high,' swallowing any statin would benefit me. Certainly, taking a statin would not spare me from a fatal heart attack or stroke."[3]

He adds, "I won't let anyone check my cholesterol until I see unequivocal data that taking a statin yields meaningful benefit for me."

That may sound like a provocative statement, to refuse to have your cholesterol levels checked, but when you look closely at the research evidence on cholesterol lowering, Dr. Hadler's opinions seem sound.

Before being screened, there's one question you have to ask yourself: Would I do anything different if the screening test showed something abnormal?

In the case of cholesterol, you might want to improve your diet, exercise more, and try to lose weight. All potentially good things, but the way your doctor may try to manage your high cholesterol will probably be by prescribing you a statin.

But how much do they help someone who is otherwise healthy? The best way to examine the evidence of the effectiveness of any drug is not by looking at single trials of that drug but by looking at what are called "meta-analyses" or overviews of the major quality studies. When you examine meta-analyses of statins, you discover that the benefits for most patients are quite small. And for some people, statins show no evidence of overall benefit whatsoever.

Such were the findings of the Therapeutics Initiative at the University of British Columbia when they did a review in 2003 of the primary prevention trials for statins (that is, trials to discover whether the drugs would prevent a heart attack in patients without established heart disease). Their meta-analysis of the five large randomized controlled trials (RCTS) of statins that had been done to that point concluded that "statins have not been shown to provide an overall health benefit in primary prevention trials."[4]

When the team updated the review in 2010,[5] they discovered that in the intervening time more RCTS had been conducted and five other systematic reviews had been published. But those reviews didn't focus on this key question: "Do the benefits of statins outweigh the harms in people with no history of heart or vascular disease?" To find the answer, the team examined an outcome called "total serious adverse events," meaning any event that led to hospitalization or death.

What the team needed to do was try to methodologically restrict the analysis to primary prevention (healthy patients) versus secondary prevention (patients who had established heart disease).

The conclusions were somewhat shocking: "Statins do not have a proven net health benefit in primary prevention populations." This means that in the settings in which they were studied, in thousands of patients over a five-year period, statins didn't reduce the overall chance of death or hospitalization.

The implications of these findings are huge, because almost all the people having their cholesterol screened, as well as about three-quarters of people currently taking statins around the world, are people like George, who have no health issues other than a failed test for cholesterol. Being labeled as having high cholesterol and swallowing a daily statin would do little to prevent them from dying or being hospitalized. They were quite likely wasting their money on the statins and quite possibly risking their health, given the potential adverse effects that come with taking any drug.

The team also found that statins have little benefit even for men who are considered high risk, such as those who have a history of heart disease plus high cholesterol. Less than 5 percent of those men would avoid having another heart attack or stroke by taking a statin every day for five years.

We've known for years that selling medication to treat your future risk for a disease is immensely profitable for the pharmaceutical industry, even when evidence of long-term health benefits is very shaky. Statin drugs are among the best-selling prescription drugs on the planet, and the pharmaceutical industry has invested heavily in convincing medical scientists, patient groups, and our prescribing doctors to think about cholesterol as a nasty foreign enemy that needs to be brought down at all costs. (In reality, cholesterol is a substance essential to life that actually resents chemical tinkering.) Cholesterol screening, therefore, is big business with big slogans and lots of money, all focused on getting people around the world to worry about their cholesterol and get it tested.

CONTROVERSY WAS writ large on the front pages of news outlets around the world in mid-November 2011 when it was reported that pediatricians at an American Heart Association conference were recommending that children as young as ages 8 or 9 should be screened for high cholesterol. Up to that point, many medical groups (such as the American Academy of Pediatrics) said that only children who are obese or have diabetes, a family history of early heart disease, or high cholesterol or high blood pressure should be screened. But with these new recommendations, they were saying that all kids needed to be screened before puberty.

This advice is bizarre, because high cholesterol isn't a disease but is a risk factor for a potential future illness—such as heart disease, which strikes mostly middle-aged and older people. Having a risk factor for a certain disease means that you might be more likely to develop that disease in the future, but that likelihood is far from certain. In fact, many people who have risk factors never go on to develop the disease in question. Furthermore, risk factors will not be present in many people who do develop the disease.

Other risk factors (such as living in poverty or being old) are much more predictive of future health problems than is the arbitrary level of cholesterol in your blood.

So why bother screening kids for a risk factor for a disease that's probably not going to hurt them for fifty, sixty, or seventy years, if ever? The answer seems to be "because we can."

The apparent rationale given at the November 2011 American Heart Association conference is that statin drugs—like Lipitor, Zocor, or Crestor—can be used "safely" in children. In addition, the experts say that with obesity on the rise in children, monitoring their cholesterol levels will only help prevent future health problems.

Some experts, though, are horrified at this expansion of cholesterol screening to children. Harriet Rosenberg is a social anthropologist at York University in Toronto and is perhaps one of Canada's foremost experts on the adverse effects of statin drugs. She finds the push to screen children for high cholesterol troubling. What is most disturbing to her is the composition of the panels that decide on who should be screened for high cholesterol.

"A healthy person is made into a patient by a blood test that is based on a consensus, of a large group of industry key opinion leaders. It's entirely sociocultural opinion."[6] And she's well aware that most of the "opinion leaders" on the panels that establish guidelines for high cholesterol have links to the pharmaceutical industry. She also finds it disquieting that the very need for cholesterol testing isn't really questioned by orthodox medicine.

All the "know your numbers" rhetoric and public exhortations to get screened, are, she says, "legitimation exercises—in other words, the more you do it, the more familiarized it becomes and the less capacity you have to ask well-informed critical questions. The public is not invited to ask why. It's in the framework of 'don't ask questions about this.'"

"Where is the demonstration that this [screening] is beneficial in some way? Or that it's cost effective? What is the story? If you have an antismoking campaign—it's pretty clear what the benefits of quitting smoking are." She goes on to ask why we wouldn't demand the same level of proof in cholesterol lowering.

Although doctors may be quick to screen patients for high cholesterol and put them on drugs to lower it, they seem to be much slower in recognizing when patients are being hurt by those drugs.

Even though the published literature is replete with case studies on the potential dangers of statins (including increased rates of kidney failure, cataracts, and serious liver and muscle damage), many physicians are unaware of even the most common side effect, which is experienced by 20 percent to 25 percent of statin-treated people: muscle pain or weakness.

The screening of our blood is perhaps so benign, so under-the-radar that we never question it. We believe that it can only do good. After all, how could one be harmed by a blood-screening test?

According to the U.S. National Heart, Lung, and Blood Institute (NHLBI), a government-funded body and part of the U.S. National Institutes of Health, "Blood tests have few risks. Most complications are minor and go away shortly after the tests are done."[7]

But the NHLBI is talking about a needle that draws blood. It's what happens afterward to that blood and how it may shape your life and your health that's the issue. What if the blood test leads to paranoia and panic in patients, an endless lifetime of worry about one's "numbers," and maybe even a steady, lifelong diet of drugs?

Many times patients submit to cholesterol or blood-sugar tests with almost no idea of what they can lead to. People like George Thompson simply trust that when they get a blood-screening test, it can only lead to good. But the inappropriate treatment of healthy people that often follows screening tests (including drugs to treat risk factors instead of real diseases) changes the equation.

The business of blood screening is extremely profitable for many players involved: the pharmaceutical industry, the physician who orders the tests and prescribes the drugs, the laboratories that do the actual tests, and the makers of home-based lab tests.

In fact, the demand for home-based lab tests is just starting to take off in an attempt to bring the patient closer to the product, cutting out the middle man. A 2011 report in the *Wall Street Journal* states that "Direct-to-consumer lab tests are a small but growing part of the overall lab industry," and also says that consumers are spending about "$20 million a year for such tests." The market for these tests is growing as much as 20 percent per year.

According to a report by Global Industry Analysts on the global cholesterol-testing market, there are three factors driving growth in the direct-to-consumer (DTC) testing market: "aging population, increasing incidence of cardiovascular diseases, and growing awareness among people about the significance of reducing the unhealthy cholesterol levels."[8]

So there you have it: the perfect storm of more boomers, more possible heart disease, and more screening.

THE SEARCH for risk factors doesn't stop with cholesterol screening. In fact, there's tremendous interest in the medical industry in screening for clusters of risk factors. Such is the case with syndrome X.

This relatively new condition is said to affect one-third of the population. According to statistics compiled by the National Health and Nutrition Examination Survey in the U.S. from 2003 to 2006, approximately 34 percent of adults in the U.S.—almost 80 million people—meet the criteria for "metabolic syndrome[9]" (also called syndrome X), which is a cluster of above-normal measurements of blood sugar, blood pressure, cholesterol, and body mass index (BMI). We are told that if you have this particular cluster of risk factors, you might be at higher risk for heart attack or stroke.

But what value is there in clustering these risk factors? Do people who wear a syndrome X label fare any better than they did before they had the label?

Good medical screening is all about discovering diseases in healthy people before those diseases can go on to hurt them. Most of us would submit to screening if we were confident it could detect disease early enough to save our lives. But how valuable is it to have a medical screening program that hunts down a collection of numbers, labels that a syndrome, and then tells us it affects one-third of the entire adult population?

As we get older, our blood pressure rises, we usually become more sedentary, and many of us get heavier. These metabolic changes may not be healthy, but for many of us, they come naturally as we get older. They are also closely linked to socioeconomic status.

But some groups (for example, those within the diabetes industry) have continued to promote the need to screen for syndrome X even though there seems to be no consensus on how to define it.[10]

Regardless of what definition you follow, a review in 2008 in the *Lancet* said that measuring syndrome X was a lousy way to determine a person's risk of future cardiovascular disease. The authors noted there are better and more accurate ways to predict cardiovascular disease and diabetes and that fasting blood sugar measurement is a cheaper and easier test and a better predictor of future diabetes than a diagnosis of metabolic syndrome.[11]

But even screening for diabetes is not without controversies.

Dr. Nortin Hadler notes that one of the main problems with screening related to diabetes is that the definitions keep changing, and what is considered a cutoff of what is "abnormal" is progressively lowered.[12] As he notes in his book *Worried Sick,* "if we keep lowering the cutoff, pretty soon all of us will age into type 2 diabetes and even more will be labeled as having the Metabolic Syndrome." He says that the "public-health world is alarming us about yet another epidemic that the pubic-health world itself is creating by virtue of changing the rules for labeling."[13]

We know that syndrome X easily fits the "more is better" ideology underlying the medical-screening paradigm, turning out more customers for pharmaceutical companies and medical lab owners. One commentator, Joanna Breitstein, writing in *PharmExec* magazine in 2004, noted that drug companies eager to sell syndrome X drugs have sponsored initiatives that emphasize the connection between insulin resistance and cardiovascular disease. She writes that that "metabolic syndrome promises to be as big as or bigger than the emergence of a market for cholesterol lowering drugs."[14]

It hasn't worked out that well, though. There have been a number of drugs specifically developed to treat syndrome X, including the drug rimonabant, an anti-obesity drug launched in Europe in 2006 and withdrawn three years later because it was linked to severe depression and suicidal thoughts. The French drug Mediator (benfluorex), a stimulant approved to treat syndrome X and type 2 diabetes but used widely in France as a weight-loss drug, was pulled off the French market in November 2010 after it was linked to as many as 2,000 deaths and many potential cases of heart valve damage.[15]

The symptoms of syndrome X are caused by both genetic and lifestyle factors, and even though you can't do much about your genes, most people are aware that the quantity and quality of food you eat and the amount of exercise you get are vital to staying healthy. And both of those factors are closely linked to your place on the socioeconomic scale, reminding us of one key, unmistakable truth: poverty is not good for your health.

Our doctors routinely screen us for obesity, hypertension, diabetes, and cholesterol. They do so in the belief that doing so will help you take action to lower your risk of heart disease. But you should be prepared to ask hard questions about what the tests might mean and what overall benefits and harms are associated with chemically altering your blood pressure, glucose, or lipid (cholesterol) levels.

A final note on syndrome X: Ironically, the physician Dr. Gerald Reaven, who coined the term syndrome X in 1988 and proposed insulin resistance as its underlying cause, later recanted. In 2006, just as the syndrome was gaining speed among the drug companies and medical authorities, he published a paper saying that physicians should stop giving this diagnosis to patients.[16]

THERE'S MONEY in screening for risk factors in your blood. But there's also plenty of cash to be made from scanning your arteries for risk as well, and that brings us to the fertile territory of heart scanning.

Even if you feel perfectly healthy, it's possible that your arteries may be so clogged that you're a walking time bomb. And the market is replete with heart and blood-vessel scanning technologies and private clinics that deliver them to paying customers.

Take, for example, Canada Diagnostic Centres' clinic in Vancouver, British Columbia, where for c$690, you can get a heart scan with Toshiba's 64-slice Aquilion CT Scanner, a high-speed, high-resolution device that can take a detailed study of "any area of the body" in seconds. The website of the Canadian Diagnostic Centres indicates that this type of heart scan (also known as coronary artery calcium scoring) would be appropriate for men aged 40 plus and women aged 50 plus.[17]

The goal of such a scan is to look for "calcified plaque build-up in the heart's arteries." Apparently, you could have such plaque and still feel fine, even do well in the standard exercise stress test and exhibit no signs of disease. Canadian Diagnostic Centres' brochure on the coronary calcium score[18] tells us that the "state-of-the-art computerized tomography methods" they employ are "the most effective way to detect early coronary calcification from atherosclerosis, before symptoms develop."

The brochure proceeds to say that "the amount of coronary calcium has been recognized as a powerful independent predictor of future cardiac events and may be used to guide lifestyle modifications and preventive medical therapies to reduce this risk."

Better safe than sorry, right? So even if you're feeling healthy, why not plunk down c$690 to determine if you have some sort of "atherosclerotic plaque." Unfortunately, many of us think of the heart's arteries as clogged plumbing and believe that all we need is a roto-rooter to get in there and clean things out. However, there is no effective drain cleaner to clean out arterial plaque.

What happens if you get a scan and it shows some plaque? The Canadian Diagnostic Centre is a little vague on that front: "This measurement, combined with your other risk factors can provide an overall picture of your heart health and can help you and your doctor develop a prevention strategy that's right for you."[19] Which is to say the recommendations that follow will likely be a litany of the usual bits of advice: change your diet and exercise habits, and possibly take some kind of preventive medication (maybe a statin?) to reduce your risk of a heart attack.

As for the c$690 cost of the heart scan, who pays for it? Will government medical plans cover it? Not likely. U.S. Medicaid and public insurers in Canada and other developed countries won't touch this type of screening with a ten-foot pole. And if public money won't pay for a particular type of medical screening, it could be because the test in question is probably of very low or unproven value and not worth covering.

But let's leave aside the question of who will pay for this scan. The real question is this: Will a coronary calcium scan of your heart save your life? Despite being widely promoted and marketed, there isn't enough evidence to say whether such screening has an overall health benefit. Again, the marketing leads and the science follows.

If you consult the screening-evidence gurus, the USPSTF, to see what they think of calcium screening, you'll find that not only do they recommend against it, the USPSTF thinks it is probably harmful. The USPSTF also recommends against three different heart screening tests: electrocardiography (ECG), exercise tread-mill testing (ETT), and electron-beam computerized tomography

(EBCT). It says that these tests should *not* be routinely done because the "harms outweigh the benefits."[20]

At the end of the day, will a heart scan lead to better health? A very interesting study in the July 2011 issue of the *Archives of Internal Medicine* found that people who had heart scans were more likely to become customers for more medications and more surgery compared with those who went the way of conventional screening. But they didn't live any longer nor were they healthier because of the scan.[21]

When I spoke to the lead author of that study, Dr. John McEvoy, he told me that there is "no difference in the health status of people who get scanned versus those who don't." Dr. McEvoy is a heart specialist and researcher at the Johns Hopkins University in Baltimore.[22]

His team examined a cohort of more than 1,000 Korean patients who got heart scans (in this case CT angiograms, a kind of 3D picture of the heart) as part of a health-screening program. His team compared these results to 1,000 closely matched individuals who just got the standard health checkup and found no difference in health status after a year and a half.

Admitting that a CT angiogram can be a very useful test in the right setting (such as when someone has chest pain or other heart symptoms), Dr. McEvoy doesn't think the evidence suggests it should be used to screen healthy people.

In fact, in his study, about 20 percent of those healthy patients who got scanned were told they had cholesterol buildup in their arteries (also called atherosclerosis) and they ended up taking a lot more drugs (aspirin and statins). The scanned patients had a lot more of everything, including more referrals for more tests, more heart bypass and stenting procedures (the insertion of tiny coils into the arteries to keep them open), and more operations. But they were no healthier after a year and a half of observation.

Acknowledging that it might take longer than eighteen months to see any effects of screening, he noted that in the short term, some patients were harmed. The scanned patients were exposed to radiation and the contrast dyes, both of which can be harmful. Excess radiation exposure may take many years to manifest, and the contrast iodine used in the screening can lead, in some cases, to kidney failure.

His conclusion: The testing might lead to more harm than good, and much of the downstream intervention and treatment in the scanned patients appeared "excessive and not necessary." Like many researchers who have closely examined the outcomes of screening, he concluded that higher quality randomized trials needed to be done to provide the conclusive proof that the scans were useful.

The practice of doing all kinds of heart scans may be discouraged by the USPSTF, but that doesn't stop physicians or private clinics from offering these services.

So what should you do?

If you're worried about heart disease, follow the lifestyle advice that most doctors and experts give: stop smoking, get regular exercise, don't eat too much fat and salt, and manage your stress. Wait a minute... isn't that the advice they give if they find you have high levels of calcium in your coronary arteries? Why yes... it is.

NO DOUBT heart disease is a big killer and hence a great concern for those who want to prevent a heart attack. Yet the examples here show that screening may do nothing to help you and may send you to the pharmacy for products that will be benign at best and harmful or potentially deadly at worse. In addition, screening for risk factors can lead to more investigations and more drugs that are widely marketed but which have little evidence to support their use.

Some screening, such as screening for specific cancers of the prostate, has been much more well studied. In the next chapter, we'll see how even the best research in the world on the pros and cons of a screening program can't always protect us from its downstream harms.

FOUR

PSA testing
What are the odds?

THE GABRIOLA Island tourist brochure says that people from Gabriola like to think of themselves as "wacky in a nice kind of way." The little community off Canada's Pacific coast is a gem of an island, nestled in coastal rain forest and only twenty minutes by ferry from the metropolis of Nanaimo. It is well known as a laid-back haven for musicians, painters, and artists of all sorts.

Musician Bob Bossin is a 65-year-old folksinger who has been a key figure in the grassroots Canadian folk music scene for decades. He is one of Gabriola's "wacky" ones, but he's also facing some big decisions. He has a form of prostate cancer that his doctors say needs to be treated but he's not sure what his best options are.

Bob sees himself as a kind of savvy poker player who knows when to hedge his bets, so when he was in his fifties and his doctor started asking him to have a digital rectal exam, he followed his doctor's advice.[1]

After the exam, his doctor said that he thought "he felt a few firmer places on the back side of the prostate." He suggested Bob go for a PSA test. After all, better safe than sorry, right?[2]

The PSA test is a simple blood test that measures the level of a substance called prostate specific antigen (PSA) and is one of the main screening tests for prostate cancer. In fact, it's used routinely to screen healthy, symptomless men for the disease, often as a part of their annual checkups. However, the PSA test is not without its problems. A "high" level of PSA can be an indicator of cancer, yet there are other conditions, such as an inflamed or enlarged prostate, that can alter one's PSA readings.

In addition to delivering false positives, the PSA test has a high incidence of false negatives. About 20 percent of men who do have prostate cancer have a normal PSA level. And if that isn't enough, the level of what's considered "normal" can be somewhat arbitrary.

What is a "normal" PSA level? In men with a perfectly healthy prostate gland, no inflammation or no cancer, the experts say the PSA reading should be less than 4 ng/Ml (nanograms per milliliter of blood). Bob's usual annual PSA score was around 4 or 5. Not really much to worry about. Yet a check in the past year had put it around 15.

Bob was sent by the urologist to get a biopsy, which involved having very fine needles inserted into the prostate (a gland about the size of a golf ball tucked above the scrotum) to get tissue samples. It's not exactly a pleasant affair, yet the twelve-snip random biopsy of Bob's prostate came back "clean as a whistle."

Obviously Bob was relieved, but with his PSA level continuing to climb, he was getting his PSA level checked about every six weeks. While the self-defined hippie tried some natural therapeutic things he'd hoped could increase his odds of keeping the PSA reading down (acupuncture, eating pomegranates, Vitamin D, and drinking green tea among others), he also took the time to educate himself about the PSA test and prostate cancer.

The first thing that men like Bob discover when they start researching prostate cancer is an adage that seems so astounding that they might disbelieve it the first time they hear it: Most men will die with prostate cancer, but not because of it.

In fact, prostate cancer is incredibly common. Men in Bob's age group have a 50 percent to 60 percent chance of having it. Yet death by it is not that common. Less than three percent of men will die from it.[3] Even though a small percent of prostate cancers are quick growing and can be rapidly lethal, most of the men who die from prostate cancers are elderly, in their seventies or eighties. With the type of low-volume, slower-growing prostate cancer that most men develop with age, it takes a long time for that cancer to become lethal, if it ever does. Often, men with this kind of prostate cancer die from something else.

Although this might seem controversial, men whose cancers are discovered as a result of a routine PSA test don't live longer than those whose cancers are discovered by other means.

Nonetheless, doctors continue to offer the PSA test annually to many of their male patients over 40, a practice recommended by the American Urological Association.[4] Other groups, such as the American Cancer Society, recommend that doctors discuss PSA testing with their male patients at age 50, particularly "men who are at average risk of prostate cancer and are expected to live at least 10 more years."[5] But there is now a growing suspicion of the whole PSA screening paradigm.

It has been building for years, but independent groups that look closely at the available evidence on screening, like the U.S. Preventive Services Task Force (USPSTF), say the PSA test simply shouldn't be done on your average man. The USPSTF's October 2011 recommendations said that the potential harms outweigh the potential benefits of PSA screening in healthy men. In particular, it said PSA screening "results in small or no reduction in prostate cancer–specific mortality and is associated with harms related to subsequent evaluation and treatments, some of which may be unnecessary."[6]

This is an astounding admission of the problems with PSA testing. Even with five well-controlled clinical trials saying that far too many men aged 50 and older are being given screening tests that won't likely help them live longer, there is high enthusiasm for PSA testing. It is estimated that 33 million U.S. men aged 50 and over (out of a total of 44 million in that age group) have already had a PSA test during their routine physical exams.

One problem is that a high PSA test gives a little bit of information but not enough. To confirm the presence of cancer, a biopsy is needed, and that is not without risk. Biopsy needles capture tiny pieces of prostate tissue and can themselves sometimes carry bacteria from the rectal wall into the prostate and bloodstream. One Canadian study found that about 4 percent of men who had prostate biopsies developed serious infections.[7] Those same numbers were confirmed by a larger 2011 study of U.S. Medicare patients undergoing biopsy, with the researchers suggesting that multidrug-resistant organisms lead to more serious complications.[8] If the infections men get from the biopsy are caused by bacteria resistant to many of the common antibiotics, those infections can seriously jeopardize the life of the patient.

A 4 percent increased risk of being hospitalized because of a prostate biopsy seems small, but not when you consider that there are more than a million or so prostate biopsies done every year in the U.S. This rate of risk could mean approximately 40,000 American males suffer biopsy-related serious infections, hospitalizations—even death—linked to infections caused by prostate biopsies.

What do the numbers say about PSA screening? In one of the largest and longest studies of the effects of PSA testing carried out in Europe, it was found that PSA testing produces a pretty small yield in terms of lives saved: A total of 1,410 men would need to be screened and 48 men would need to be treated to save one life. Of the other 47 treated men—sometimes with surgery, chemotherapy, and drugs—many would be left impotent or incontinent.[9] As one doctor once joked to me, after being treated for prostate cancer, you may not live longer, but your life will *feel* longer.

There are many ways to treat prostate cancer, including hormone drugs, chemotherapy, radical prostatectomy (where the prostate is surgically removed), brachytherapy (radioactive pellets inserted into the tumor), cryotherapy (freezing the tumor), and what is known as "watchful waiting."

Watchful waiting may very well be the most difficult option for most men, but it is a viable course of action *because most of the time, nothing bad will happen.* The fact is that the vast majority of prostate cancers are the slow-growing type. But watching and waiting goes against the best instincts of many of us who would say, "I've got cancer? Okay, doc, go ahead, do whatever cutting and chemo you need to do to get rid of it."

Unfortunately, what most men really need when faced with the array of treatments available is some sense of which one works best. The needed evidence, however, is sparse. The internationally renowned Cochrane Collaboration (Cochrane.org) could only find two randomized controlled trials[10] that compared watchful waiting to radical prostatectomy (in patients who had symptoms) and couldn't say with any certainty which worked better. The higher quality, Scandinavian study[11] over twelve years found that overall death rates were lower with radical prostatectomy for men under 65 but not for men over 65. The authors conclude that there wasn't enough evidence to make confident statements about which treatment was superior.[12]

What is known is that men who undergo surgery have a higher chance of becoming impotent or incontinent. A 2000 study looked at men who underwent radical prostatectomy, randomly sampled from six National Cancer Institute cancer registries across the United States. It found that 60 percent of the men were impotent 18 months after the surgery and 8 percent had urinary incontinence.[13]

Given the inconclusiveness of whether treatment leads to a better result than just watching and waiting, what's a man to do? Even a man like Bob Bossin, who has read many books, consulted experts, and is highly literate on the subject, is left with many unanswered questions as to what he should do next, since a diagnosis of cancer has now been confirmed by a second biopsy. However, he believes that waiting and seeing is not for him. Since he has lost friends to prostate cancer, he doesn't want to take that chance.

But there are other men who know all the data and choose to watch and wait. Calvin Cairns, 57, is one of Bob Bossin's friends, a fiddling genius who lives in Victoria, British Columbia. He used to tour with Bob in the 1980s as part of a folk music group called Stringband. Like Bob, Calvin Cairns had his PSA tested, and was told it was "high." He went on to have a biopsy that confirmed a diagnosis of prostate cancer.

He now refers to that diagnosis as a turning point in his life, one which led him to embark on a spiritual journey and a major re-evaluation of his life. "It really brought my mortality to the fore," he said. In the end, he was glad that such an event forced him to reconnect with his spiritual side.[14]

But before he could reap that benefit, he first had to deal with the demands of the medical system. His doctor, he said, "leaned on me pretty hard to go for a radical prostatectomy."

Calvin started doing his research. He says that once he "got over the shock" of his diagnosis and started educating himself about prostate cancer, he realized that a person of his age with his diagnosis fit into a "large gray area."

In fact, as he dug deeper into the research, he discovered that the aggressive treatments—like prostate surgery—that men are pushed toward here in North America were "way more radical than what would happen in Europe." In other words, he realized that there were cultural dimensions to treating his particular state of prostate cancer and that a radical prostatectomy probably wouldn't have been recommended for a patient like him if he lived in Europe.

He amassed as much information as he could, met with alternative medical practitioners, and ultimately decided that aggressive treatment was not for him. He has chosen to wait and see.

One of the hardest parts for him was not letting his fear override his intuition. Ultimately, taking the option of "watchful waiting" made him look for what else he could do to stay healthy and grounded. He admits that researching the various ways prostate cancer is treated drove him to seek out the low-tech, non-invasive, "alternative" options out there.

Despite the confusing array of options facing men who have been through the PSA mill—and despite authoritative organizations like the USPSTF saying that not only does the test offer little to no reduction in mortality rates, but also that some of the subsequent evaluations and treatments that follow a high PSA test may be unnecessary—the PSA screening juggernaut seems to plow on, oblivious to one key problem that faces anyone getting not just a PSA test, but any screening test: Once it's done, you can't "unknow" what you know. A seed has been planted either of doubt or certainty.

There is no doubt that the standard prostate screening tools (PSA testing and digital rectal exams) are an ingrained part of medical culture. The supposed benefits of these tests are seized upon with hope and optimism, whereas the adverse effects are ignored or downplayed. The stories of men who claim to have had their lives "saved" by PSA testing are certainly more shared and retold than the stories of men left impotent or incontinent. And these things have kept the PSA test and general "prostate awareness" activities alive. There is a name for this phenomenon—the popularity paradox—coined by Muir Gray and Angela Raffle in their book *Screening: Evidence and Practice."* The authors say this: "The greater the overdiagnosis and overtreatment, the more people there are who believe they owe their health or even their life to the programme."[15]

Some "prostate awareness" projects are problematic, however. An enormous amount of corporate money is thrown at cancer fundraisers around the world every year. One organization whose slickness is an easy reminder of how much corporate money it's soaking in is Zero: The Project to End Prostate Cancer (ZeroCancer.org).

The Zero folks have set themselves an incredibly lofty goal: "We're committed to creating Generation Zero: the first generation of men free from prostate cancer," their website proclaims. One of their key messages: Get a PSA test.

And Zero likes to make it easy for men to get that test. One of their campaign arms asks, "Can't get where you need to go for a PSA test? Then join Zero's Drive Against Prostate Cancer." According to its site, "More than 110,000 men have been tested for free onboard the Drive Against Prostate Cancer mobile medical program since 2002. From tracking high PSA test results and then alerting those men to see their doctor, the Drive has saved as many as 12,000 lives."

Like a lot of male-dominated disease groups, the leadership at Zero know that men—certainly in Canada, anyway—are obsessed with hockey, and Zero's website makes the rather bizarre claim that Zero is the "The Official Prostate Cancer Charity of the National Hockey League."

Zero also has a serious political side to its activities. Just as the USPSTF was updating its recommendations on PSA testing in November 2011, Zero jumped into action. It began lobbying the U.S. Congress to make sure that no one could take away men's god-given right to wear diapers.

Diapers? Yes. In part of a press release announcing that "ZERO Works with Congress to Protect Early Detection," the organization said it was mounting an "aggressive campaign on Capitol Hill to combat the task force's infringement on the doctor-patient relationship."[16] One of their corporate partners in this effort is Depends, a brand of adult diapers (Depends.com). The makers of Depends are also unafraid of jumping into the ring to participate in what seems like fearmongering around prostate cancer. Depends says, "Every three minutes a man in this country finds out he has prostate cancer. The good news is that early detection (a result of screening!) comes with an almost 100% survival rate."[17]

Depends' website reminds us that "Depend® brand has teamed up with ZERO, the project to end prostate cancer, to help get the word out about prostate health."[18]

Who is benefiting from all this testing? Clearly the major beneficiaries of PSA screening and the biggest supporters of keeping it alive are the ones who profit most from treating it: drug companies, urologists, and radiation therapists.

Compared to the cost of treatment, the testing itself is inexpensive. Nonetheless, with more than 30 million PSA tests performed annually in the U.S. alone,[19] that market is worth about $1 billion annually.[20] One company, Mediwatch, is distributing worldwide its point-of-care PSA measuring system called PSAwatch, which would help move PSA testing from diagnostic labs to physicians' offices. The appeal is that the money currently going to the labs would be staying in physicians' bank accounts.[21] But how, exactly, would doctors be able to have an informed conversation with a patient on PSA testing if they stand to profit from it? Wouldn't it be hard to be an advocate for your patient when you're getting money by testing them?

The "prostate cancer cauldron" represents "a multibillion-dollar industry," according to medical oncologist, Dr. Mark Scholz.[22]

To answer the question of who benefits from PSA testing, he says that you have to follow the money. Dr. Mark Scholz is the medical director of a prostate cancer clinic in Marina del Ray, California, and he co-wrote (with journalist Ralph Blum) *The Invasion of the Prostate Snatchers*. What motivated him to write this book was that he "absolutely abhorred . . . the rolling disaster that no one seems to want to do anything about."

He says that most cancer treatment in the U.S. is managed by oncologists (specialists in cancer) but prostate cancer treatment is managed by urologists—who are surgeons.

In Dr. Scholz's estimation, the "PSA is like bait to put out for animals to suck them into the gravitational pull of the surgeons, who immediately cut their prostate out."

Those are harsh words, but there are data to back them up.

"Even though in the last five years they realized that you can safely watch about a third of newly diagnosed men," he says, "the use of surgery has almost doubled."

"What's that about?" I asked him.

His rapid-fire explanation comes in two words: "Robotic surgery." High-tech computers are brought in to do the surgery. Dr. Scholz is dismissive, calling it just "another type of surgery… The robotic part is a bit of a misnomer; they have a human that is steering the thing." Is it better to be operated on by a robot? Not really. The rates of incontinence and impotence are similar to conventional surgery, and there is no long-term evidence on the effectiveness of robotic prostate surgery.

He reckons that going even higher tech is good for business and attractive to patients. The robotic surgery on men's prostates "is so exciting to the surgeons, they're scooping up even more people to operate on… It's a shocking situation."

And there is evidence that hospitals that require surgical robots carry out many more radical prostatectomies than those that don't. The underlying issue here is that hospitals may be able to increase their revenues by carrying out more robotic surgeries.[23]

Prostate snatchers indeed.

Dr. Scholz's bottom line is that patients need to be educated. He stresses that the "field is so complex, if you don't educate yourself you'll end up making big mistakes."

One man who has spent many years thinking about and studying medical screening and the value of PSA testing is Dr. H. Gilbert Welch, co-author (with Steve Woloshin and Lisa Schwartz) of *Overdiagnosed: Making People Sick in the Pursuit of Health.* He admits that it's difficult to quantify the benefits and harms of prostate cancer screening but estimates, given currently available data, that "for every man who benefits from screening by avoiding a prostate cancer death, somewhere between thirty and a hundred are harmed by overdiagnosis and treated needlessly."[24]

And here is a difficult thought to process: If prostate screening resulted only in treatment that was justified (and led to a longer and healthier life, for example), those doing the treating would likely lose most of their work.

Whether we like it or not, urologists have an unavoidable conflict of interest regarding PSA screening because if so much of their work depends on treating prostate cancer when they see it, it is hard for them to be critical of PSA testing. In fact, asking a urologist if you need a PSA test or if you need surgery to treat what a biopsy has found might be like asking your barber if you need a haircut. You are asking the right question of the wrong person.

Then there are those who supply the radiation, says Dr. Scholz. He notes that since "radiation therapists are highly remunerated to radiate prostates, there is a lot of unnecessary radiation going on."

And Dr. Scholz says that in the U.S. they do very well with prostate radiation. "They get $40,000 to radiate one prostate." He goes on to wonder aloud, "There's a little bit of incentive there." It doesn't sound like terribly hard work either, as he scoffs, "You line 'em up and turn them over to your radiation technician and collect the cash."

Then there's the drug industry. According to Decision Resources, an advisory firm that analyzes developments in the pharmaceutical and health-care industry, several launches of new prostate cancer therapies will increase the size of the market from $3.6 billion in 2010 to $10.1 billion in 2020 in seven major industrialized countries.[25]

It has been only recently that the value of the PSA test has come under serious scrutiny, with debates being played out in the public sphere. Dr. H. Gilbert Welch sums up the situation in one simple soundbite: The PSA test is the "poster child for overdiagnosis."

This assessment is echoed by Richard Ablin, whose opinion about the PSA test might be worth listening to as he is the scientist credited with its discovery in 1970. Writing in the *New York Times* in March 2010, Ablin said, "The test's popularity has led to a hugely expensive public health disaster. It's an issue I am painfully familiar with."[26]

Despite all the problems with PSA screening tests, there is still a very strong belief in the value of surveillance, in being ever-vigilant to the possibility of disease.

In practice, it's easy for doctors to recommend patients for tests, and writing out the order is much less difficult than having the long discussion patients really need to make an informed decision about the test. One survey of physicians in an East Coast HMO found that doctors ordered PSA testing an average of 81 percent of the time for their asymptomatic male patients over age 50, but less than half of those doctors believed "that aggressive early treatment of prostate cancer improved patient outcomes."[27] The survey left me with an obvious question: If many of these doctors don't believe that early detection improves outcomes, why are they ordering so many tests?

It's a very good question with no precise or easy answer.

Do they order tests because they are afraid of being sued? Because they believe their patients expect it? Because it is considered the "standard of practice"? Because their peers do it and they don't want to be perceived as out of line with their peers?[28] All of these factors might be in play, but what about those on the receiving end of the test?

Do patients actually want the tests? Do they see every test as only being beneficial? One theory is that if evidence is presented that favors a test, it is more likely to be absorbed than evidence against a test. A Michigan study looked at men's attitudes after they had been given educational, objective counseling about the PSA test's various benefits and risks. Even though 90 percent thought the information presented to them was unfavorable toward PSA testing, many rejected the information because it didn't fall in line with their own beliefs.[29] This phenomenon is called "confirmation bias" and refers to the tendency to give more attention to data that support our beliefs and ignore data that contradict our beliefs.

In the Michigan study, of the 40 men interviewed, 29 of 30 who had been screened before continued to want future screening. One might have summed up the collective feeling of the cohort by saying: "If there's a test, or an exam, or something, I'm going to take it."

Calvin Cairns's own diagnosis with prostate cancer has resulted in him taking a "watchful waiting" approach. Even though his life has been turned upside down by this diagnosis, he remains enthusiastic about the PSA test. I asked him if he would recommend it to people like me in middle age who had never had one.

"Absolutely," he says. "You need to know what your baseline is."

He goes on to say, "In my experience it has been very useful—it sent the flag up, got me turned around, led me to an early diagnosis, and enabled me to make changes in my life."

But he has one caveat: He wouldn't recommend any man get a PSA test without first educating himself about the disease. "You need to be aware of the disease so when you get the PSA test, it won't knock you off balance. You need to be grounded in knowledge. You have to enter it from that perspective, instead of the one of fear and ignorance."

Despite all the controversies around PSA testing between those promoting it and those trying to rein things in, the fiddler Calvin Cairns has hit the right note when it comes to the one solid and indisputable commonality: Men need to go into prostate screening with their eyes wide open. If they are going to have a screening test such as this—which could radically change their lives—they need to agree to it only after a full assessment of the possible good, the bad, and the ugly of PSA testing. Perhaps the best way to start is to read a reasonably good and informative factsheet, like the one produced by the National Cancer Institute in the U.S., and prepare yourself for the inevitable discussion with your doctors.[30] Another brilliant resource is chapter 4, "We Look Harder for Prostate Cancer," in Dr. H. Gilbert Welch's *Overdiagnosed*.

And think about your odds. Above all, it is worth avoiding information that comes from surgery clinics, prostate cancer advocacy groups, professional associations, and others who might have conflicts of interest about finding and treating cancer and hence could deliver biased recommendations.

Bob Bossin's diagnosis is interfering with his current project: writing a book about his father, who was a prominent figure in the gambling business in the 1930s and 1940s in eastern Canada. Bob, a veteran recreational poker player, now finds himself in a game where the stakes are life and death. But as every poker player knows, you have to play the hand you are dealt. "If I play my cards right, I could win another twenty years," he muses philosophically, "if not..."

Has modern medicine overpromised when it comes to men like Bob Bossin or Calvin Cairns, claiming that screening will save them from prostate cancer deaths? Undoubtedly, it has. Perhaps now is the time to balance out those promises with a new mindset: Let no man submit to a PSA test until he is aware of the game, his odds, the size of the pot, and how the deck might be stacked against him.

FIVE

Mammography screening

The politics, the promises, and the numbers

MARY BROWN (not her real name) is an educator in Vancouver who underwent her first and only screening mammogram a few years ago.

She said that her doctor wasn't pressuring her. "My doctor inquired about my history and asked if I'd had a mammogram. She said maybe I don't need to think about this 'til I'm 50. It wasn't on my mind. But with more and more people getting cancer... Father, office workers, and so on getting cancer..."[1]

So when Mary was wrapping up her father's estate, the idea of going for a mammogram came up. She was chatting with relatives and friends at her dad's funeral, and several women aired their personal views about breast cancer screening. She found that there was a kind of excitement around it. "People really encouraged me to go," she said. So she did.

Two years later, including eight months off work dealing with chronic pain, occasional panic attacks, and the lingering side effects from a breast biopsy, she calls that mammogram "the biggest mistake of my life."

Like many people who have faced medical adversity, pain, and loss through standard orthodox medicine, Mary has become a fierce advocate for women's right to know everything they should know about breast cancer screening *before* they agree to it.

For Mary, the most striking thing was what she wasn't told.

"There wasn't much information available—even the people working there don't know much about the procedures," she says. "All the literature, the invitation letters welcoming you to participate [in the screening program] seemed so benign. There was no hint of possible harm."

Mary was told that the biopsy might involve "mild discomfort," and she says "the word 'pain' wasn't even mentioned."

"I asked about nerve damage. I asked specific questions about this. And it was flatly denied that there was any pain or nerve damage involved."

What Mary discovered is that during the biopsy to extract tissue samples, a metal marker might be implanted in the breast and left there permanently.

"It's part of breast-conservation therapy. It's so if you have surgery, they can more easily locate the site in surgery… It's so they can find it."

Mary is concerned that many women may not be aware that a breast biopsy that leaves metal implanted in the breast tissue can cause some women extreme and long-lasting pain as well as internal scarring, not to mention the psychological effects of having a potentially disfigured breast.

What made Mary so angry wasn't that her biopsy ended up causing her severe pain and disability, but that the mammography screening program kept her in the dark on what to expect. Her experience highlights an important aspect of mammography, one that has been at the heart of the breast cancer screening debate for years: the issue of informed consent.

Mary followed up her experience with a complaint to the local college of physicians and surgeons, the body that regulates the province's physicians, focusing on problems resulting from the lack of information on the potential downside of the screening mammogram. She concludes that most women will be unaware, as she was, of the problems of the mammogram, and says, "They are marketing a potentially harmful screening test."

Her situation may be an anomaly, but how often do breast biopsies cause harm? How often are women hurt—or helped—by the very act of breast cancer screening? While screening for breast cancer might be harmful for some, is it still saving lives?

Those questions are at the heart of a serious global debate that pits survivors, advocates, and many within the breast cancer establishment against those who have looked hard at the numbers from quality randomized trials and come to the same conclusion that Mary Brown did: that there is a lot of misinformation swirling around breast cancer screening.

Perhaps nothing highlights this debate more than when national task forces change their recommendations on who should be screened, when, and how often. Such was the case in November 2011 when the Canadian Task Force on Preventive Health Care put forward a new set of mammography recommendations. The new guidelines said that routine screening of women should not begin until age 50, and that women between 40 and 49 should not be screened for breast cancer. This was a change from an earlier (2001) guideline that said that "upon reaching the age of 40 Canadian women should be informed of the potential benefits and risks of screening mammography and assisted in deciding at what age they wish to initiate the manoeuvre."[2]

A front-page story in USA Today, one of the largest circulation newspapers in the U.S., on November 21, 2011, was perhaps typical of the massive amount of media attention attracted by Canada's new recommendations. The bold headline stated, "Canadian Guidelines Support No Routine Mammograms until 50."[3]

But the idea of age 50 as the time to begin screening wasn't exactly new; the same recommendation had been made two years previously by the U.S. equivalent of Canada's task force, the U.S. Preventive Services Task Force (USPSTF). When the USPSTF said that women should be routinely screened at 50, virtually every big media outlet in the U.S., including the *Wall Street Journal*, the *Washington Post*, and the *New York Times*, reported on the firestorm of controversy that resulted.

The power of the breast cancer lobby and the accompanying media-fueled controversy caused the U.S. Health and Human Services Secretary Kathleen Sebelius to back away from the recommendation.

One finds a common strain of attack among those who criticize the guidelines. The government advisory bodies are only trying to save money by restricting screening. This idea, however, is a red herring, as neither the Canadian nor the American task forces took into account the economics of screening in preparing their guidelines.

Many pro-screening advocates believe that cutting or restricting screening means women will die. A September 2011 poll of American voters found that "nearly 90 percent of women who had a mammogram considered mammograms important to their health and well-being."[4]

Canada's task force recommended against routine screening mammography in women aged 40 to 49 years and suggested that women between 50 and 74 should be screened only every two or three years. One thing that the recent changes to the Canadian guidelines made clear is that society's conceptions of the value of mammography are undergoing a big rethink.

Mammographic screening of the breasts uses X-rays to discover masses that could be breast cancer. If detected early, it is believed, small tumors (the ones you can't yet feel) can be found, tested, and removed before they become bigger and spread to other organs.

It's important to make the distinction that population screening is strictly about doing mammograms on women who have no symptoms. When a woman does have symptoms of breast cancer (a lump or something else unusual), she receives a diagnostic mammogram.

Behind the changing recommendations is an accumulation of evidence that there are considerable harms associated with widespread mammography screening and that the benefits are a lot more modest than previously thought.

One researcher who has helped accumulate this evidence is Dr. Cornelia Baines, a physician-epidemiologist and researcher at the Dalla Lana School of Public Health at the University of Toronto. She has carried out one of the world's best studies on breast cancer screening, the "Canadian National Breast Screening Study" (CNBSS). For more than two decades, she has been involved in the controversies over the evidence and has witnessed a lifetime of criticism leveled against those like her who choose to cast a critical—one might say, more evidence-based—eye on screening.

The breast cancer screening industry is a huge business. In the U.S., about $5 billion per year is spent carrying out an estimated 48 million annual mammograms. Like any big business, the financial interests of powerful medical device makers; influential medical professionals (radiologists, pathologists, and surgeons); and funded patient groups are harnessed to the same ox, pulling usually in the same direction: more, not less, screening. The mantras are worn clichés: *Early detection will save your life. Get screened. Do it for the ones you love.*

The screening market is, in part, buoyed by the motivations of physicians and lawyers. We tend to punish physicians for sins of omission, not sins of commission. If a physician doesn't offer the patient a screening test, and that patient later gets sick or even dies because of the disease that she should have been screened for, is a lawsuit warranted? Also, the fear of missing something strongly motivates radiologists to err on the side of caution and bring attention to every little lump and abnormality they find. After all, anything could look like cancer. The influence of the legal system in screening is unavoidable, and one study found that the most common reason that radiologists in Europe and the U.S. find themselves facing malpractice cases is for allegedly missing an abnormality in a mammography exam.[5]

Dr. Baines has seen screening advocates direct their ire against the government-appointed task forces, both in Canada and the U.S., when those panels come up with disagreeable conclusions—such as the need to be more selective in who is screened and the reality that more screening presents more overall harms to women. She wrote in 2005, "I remain convinced that the current enthusiasm for screening is based more on fear, false hope, and greed than on evidence."[6]

The general public may not be aware of the potential for strong financial conflicts of interest in the screening world. Those speaking and publicly promoting screening (radiologists, surgeons, and patient advocates) often have financial interests in what they recommend, and those interests aren't brought forward to a media-consuming audience.

Many of us probably know of women who have had a mammogram that found "something suspicious," possibly a cancer. Regardless of what happened next, they may feel that their lives were spared. And those who survive the ordeal that follows, or who are close to someone who has, often become volunteer footsoldiers in the war on breast cancer. Those foot soldiers are quick to defend the screening test as obviously, and profoundly, lifesaving and are quick to criticize those who question it. Dr. Baines has been on the receiving end of a lot of public invective and has also heard of a lot of nasty behavior deployed against those who question screening, including "threatening phone calls, and in one instance, the physical attack of a chairwoman of a U.K. panel discussion on screening."

As an epidemiologist, Dr. Cornelia Baines agrees that the lack of understanding (or perhaps self-deception) about the numbers makes people believe mammography is much more effective and less harmful than it actually is. It is therefore important to look closely at the numbers related to breast cancer screening.

We'll look at three distinct and commonly quoted numbers:

The rate of reduction in breast cancer
deaths due to mammography screening

Most cancer agencies and advocacy groups working in breast cancer stress that early detection is the best way to avoid death from breast cancer. The claims made regarding how much women will benefit from mammography screening vary. For example, the National Cancer Institute in the U.S. states that "research shows that screening mammography helps reduce the number of deaths from breast cancer among women ages 50 to 74 by about 17 percent."[7] The Canadian Breast Cancer Foundation[8] says that "mammography has been widely tested and proven to help reduce deaths from breast cancer by 25–35 per cent in women who start screening by mammography from the age of 40."[9]

It's hard to be precise as to what the effectiveness of a screening mammography program actually is, but let's assume it reduces mortality from breast cancer by somewhere between 17 percent to 35 percent. What does that mean?

Reducing something by a certain percent makes no sense unless you know the number from which it is being reduced. In this case, we need to know how many unscreened women die from breast cancer before we can determine the magnitude of life-saving benefits due to screening.

Here it's useful to think of two populations of women who are the same except that one group gets screened annually—in this case, 2,000 women who are screened annually for 10 years and 2,000 women who are not.

If 2,000 women over age 50 undergo annual mammography screening for 10 years, let's say there will be 3 women who die from breast cancer. Of the 2,000 women who don't get the screening, there will be 4 women who die. This is called the absolute benefit: 1 woman in 2,000 has had her life saved from screening over 10 years. Another way to look at this is to see that 3 is "25 percent less than" 4. So if screening reduces your risk of death from 4 to 3, that's a drop of 25 percent. But it's really only 1 in 2,000 women who has benefited.

Do you think those statistics are a bit deceptive? Luckily, there are some great tools to prevent you from being bamboozled by health statistics, including an excellent book by Drs. Lisa Schwartz, Steve Woloshin, and H. Gilbert Welch titled *Know Your Chances: Understanding Health Statistics.*[10]

Let's be clear: Most cancer advocacy groups make screening sound attractive by expressing the benefits of mammography in similar "relative" risk reductions. But remember this any time someone throws impressive statistics your way: Learning that a new pair of pants is "25% off the regular price!" is not that helpful unless you know the price they were to start with.

So when you hear that screening produces a 25 percent reduction in breast cancer mortality or 17 percent or 40 percent, you need to ask, "Of what?" What is the real, absolute risk to start with? How many women do you need to screen to save one life?

The new recommendation from the Canadian Task Force on Preventive Health Care expressed the benefits this way: "Screening about 2,100 women aged 40–49 years once every 2–3 years for about 11 years would prevent a single death from breast cancer."[11]

So with a one in 2,100 chance of having your life saved, you have to ask, what else happens along the way?

The rate of overdiagnosis due to mammography screening

Like many screening programs, one of the key problems with screening for breast cancer is overdiagnosis. Sometimes what may appear to be a deadly cancer isn't cancer at all. Slight lesions in milk ducts in a woman's breasts may look cancerous, and finding them on a mammogram may lead to a cascade of anxiety, further investigations, biopsies, surgery, and drugs, even if they would never have gone on to hurt the woman.

Dr. H. Gilbert Welch, author of the book *Overdiagnosed: Making People Sick in the Pursuit of Health,* is a well-known authority on the subject of cancer overdiagnosis.

In the *Journal of the National Cancer Institute,* he and his co-author William Black wrote that overdiagnosis occurs when "either nonprogressive cancers or very slow-growing cancers (more precisely, at a slow enough pace that individuals die from something else before the cancer ever causes symptoms) are detected."[12]

Together, they call these two forms of cancer "pseudodisease"; literally, false disease. The big problem is that often physicians cannot distinguish between the overdiagnosed and those requiring treatment.

When the two researchers looked closely at randomized trials, they estimated that overdiagnosis occurs in "about 25% of mammographically detected breast cancers, 50% of chest X-ray and/or sputum-detected lung cancers, and 60% of prostate-specific antigen-detected prostate cancers."[13]

A meta-analysis produced by researchers at the Cochrane Collaboration and published in the BMJ pegged mammography overdiagnosis a bit higher, saying that "one in three breast cancers detected in a population offered organised screening is overdiagnosed."[14]

As mentioned above, screening over 2,100 women for 11 years may prevent one death from breast cancer, but not without harm. According to the Canadian Task Force, screening that many women for that long would result "in about 690 women having a false-positive result on a mammogram, leading to unnecessary follow-up testing, and 75 women having an unnecessary biopsy of their breast."[15]

It goes without saying that a benign "false scare" can put a woman on an emotional roller coaster. She may end up on a medical treadmill that may involve, among other things, medical appointments and psychotherapeutic drugs such as antidepressants, as well as the anxiety, worry, stress, and time away from family. She becomes a "cancer patient" living under a cloud because the biopsy may be just the beginning of numerous other problems.

Just ask Mary Brown what she thinks of the information given to women prior to having a biopsy. Is it adequate? Probably not.

But this brings us to another number.

The drop in the number of breast cancer deaths overall in the past 15 years

Between 1995 and 2010, the death rate from breast cancer in the U.S. went from 33.1 per 100,000 to 24 per 100,000, where it roughly stands today. There is no doubt that the drop in breast cancer deaths is a sign of progress made in the fight against this particular cancer during the last 15 years. In Canada, similar figures are reported, with the Canadian Cancer Society saying that Canada's "breast cancer death rate has declined by more than 25% since 1986."[16]

Almost all the literature you'll read on the reductions in breast cancer deaths in the last few decades mention that the reductions are due to screening programs.

However, it's not that simple.

At the end of July 2011, a study published in the BMJ led by a team of researchers from Norway, France, and the U.K. found that "breast cancer screening has not played a direct part in the reductions of breast cancer mortality in recent years."[17] The researchers say that improved health systems and better treatments are more likely the cause of reduced numbers of breast cancer deaths.

Dr. Cornelia Baines also says the reductions seen in breast cancer deaths cannot be due to screening. She notes that "improvements in therapy (such as chemo- and hormone therapy) since the 1980s, when many screening trials were conducted, have undoubtedly contributed to the breast cancer mortality reduction observed in both screened and unscreened women."[18] And there's another fact that is seldom scrutinized: The drop in breast cancer is partly due to the substantial reductions in the amount of hormone replacement therapy taken by menopausal women since 2003.

At the end of the day, what's a woman to do?

Individually, it is hard not to want to do everything you can do to avoid death by breast cancer, and a mammogram seems a small price to pay. We might hope for the best, believe what the advocates and promoters of breast cancer screening say, but at the end of the day, the numbers may send a different message. And those numbers tend to take the wind out of the sails of those pushing for more and more mammography screening.

The scholar Devra Davis, an epidemiologist and president of the Environmental Health Trust, pointed out in her excellent book *The Secret History of the War on Cancer,* "The marketing of mammography, ultrasound and breast MRI seems to have a life of its own, where the opportunity to conduct hard, cold analysis is hamstrung by the fabulous profitability of the business."[19]

When money is involved, money will shape the debate.

But only if we let it.

If we were really concerned with saving lives and minimizing harm to women, we'd do much better as a society in creating and then listening to the most objective science. We'd disseminate understandable numbers to people in the clearest, most unbiased manner possible. We'd demand clearer answers about the pluses and minuses of mammography, and we'd protest the lack of quality information about potential harms. We wouldn't weasel around trying to attribute reductions in breast cancer to screening or pressure women into thinking that their choice not to be screened is irrational.

This is not an easy task given the strong "screen early and screen often" message that characterizes public discussion. The public might be bombarded with stories of women who say their lives have been saved by a screening mammogram, but it's time to tell also the stories of women who have been overdiagnosed.

Perhaps Cornelia Baines said it best, referring to the risks of overdiagnosis and harms related to breast screening: "After over 20 years of involvement in the screening controversy, I can only conclude that this is information few want to hear and many want to suppress."[20]

SIX

Colon and cervix screening
Too much of a good thing?

IT WAS supposed to be a simple routine colon scan.

The patient was Dr. William Casarella,[1] professor of radiology at Emory University School of Medicine in Atlanta, and the scan he got was not unlike the kind that he, as a doctor, had carried out on hundreds of his own patients.

Nonetheless, that scan began an adventure that ended in major surgery. He described himself waking up in the recovery room after five hours of surgery, "with a chest tube, a Foley catheter, a subclavian central venous catheter, a nasal oxygen catheter, an epidural catheter, an arterial catheter, subcutaneously administered heparin, a constant infusion of prophylactic antibiotics, and patient-controlled analgesia with intravenously administered narcotics."[2]

What was going on? Dr. Casarella was lying in a hospital bed, with needles all over his body and tubes carrying drugs, painkillers, and anesthetics into his veins, and more tubes leaving his body draining other fluids. He also had a massive scar down the middle of his chest. He had just undergone a thoracotomy, a major operation on his chest.

All this medical activity had started months before, with a simple CT scan of his colon. What had gone wrong?

Dr. Casarella had spent a professional lifetime screening and diagnosing people with disease. One of the key tasks of radiologists is interpreting the images of organs that emerge from high-tech machines such as CT scanners or MRI devices. Certainly as someone who screens patients for a living, Dr. Casarella was well versed in the pros and cons of screening for cancer in the colon.

But perhaps because he had access to the highest of high-tech devices, he opted to undergo a CT screening test: a "virtual colonoscopy." Of course, he had other options available to him, but a CT scan, which uses radiation to take hundreds of virtual "slices" of the organ in question, is highly sensitive. If there is any procedure on the planet that is capable of finding abnormalities in the colon, it's going to be a virtual colonoscopy.

Dr. Casarella's colon scan, however, was not isolated to just the colon. It also captured part of his lungs, his kidneys, his liver, and other internal organs. It found potential abnormalities on several of the organs surrounding his colon. And one of those abnormalities, on his lungs, led to major surgery.

Colon cancer screening and cervical cancer screening are both categorized as "recommended and likely helpful." However, research and experience has found that although such screening can deliver benefits, their widespread use on a symptomless population has the potential for serious consequences. Caution is always a useful watchword when it comes to screening, and screening for colon and cervical cancers is no exception.

THE COLON is a nearly six-foot-long tube that makes up much of the large intestine as it snakes its way across your abdomen, absorbing nutrients, minerals, and water along the way and literally moving out the crap your body doesn't need.

But because it is such an active organ, the colon can cause a significant amount of disease. Colorectal cancer is the third most common type of cancer in both men and women in the United States. Overall cancer deaths have been declining since the 1990s, but colorectal cancer still strikes about 150,000 Americans per year and about a third of those will die from it.[3]

Colon cancer is not something to be trifled with, and so it's not surprising that routine colon screening—through a variety of methods—is recommended. There's a menu of options for you to consider, ranging from the simple (but yucky, and perhaps somewhat imprecise) fecal occult blood test, where a stool sample is sent to a lab for analysis, to a flexible sigmoidoscopy, to a regular colonoscopy. Those last two are more invasive procedures that involve some level of anesthetics and probing up the rectum with various cameras and tools.

Or you could do as Dr. Casarella did, and opt for the virtual colonoscopy, deemed to be less invasive as it doesn't involve probing. In 2002, in *Radiology*, one of the most prestigious medical journals read by his profession, Dr. Casarella published a short letter describing his experience, with the preamble that "what is often missing from radiologists' thoughts is firsthand experience with the clinical drama that follows screening or diagnostic tests."

Dr. Casarella showed a generosity of spirit and patience when I interviewed him about his experience. He said that what "a lot of individuals who talk about using imaging for screening don't usually mention is that you find other things. The CT scan, of course, takes slices through the entire body, so it's not limited to the colon. You do see the kidneys, the liver, the base of the lungs, and so on."[4]

He went on to describe the potential downside to the kind of scan he had, saying, "You can find unexpected fortuitous findings that could be important but [could be] also very misleading. In my case, there were multiple lesions." In a nutshell, the scanner found all kinds of things in his body that may have looked like cancer and so required a closer examination.

Dr. Casarella is aware that his experience almost makes him the poster child for colon screening overdiagnosis, and he uses a royal sounding "we" when he talks about what the scan found inside his body. He explains: "We had a renal kidney mass—turned out to be a cyst. We had to interrogate the kidney with another scan with contrast to prove it was a benign cyst. There were a couple of areas that were questionable in the liver—those wound up undergoing a liver biopsy that proved to be not significant. There were a couple of masses on the base of a lung. It was difficult to tell with the lung. It's hard to be 100 percent sure if it is a malignancy, a metastatic problem from another site, a residual from an old infection, a little granuloma."

There's a useful analogy here. If you look at your arms and legs closely, you'll find scars, scabs, bumps, moles, and weird bits of flesh that you've acquired throughout your life. Your skin is like a road map of the wounds and experiences of your past. Maybe it's that bike accident when you were 12, or a birthmark you were born with, or a scar on your thumb from an old incident with a fishhook. But just as all that happens on the outside of our bodies, we've got the same internal markers inside us. Our internal organs carry signs of many of our past adventures: the scars, lesions, and nodules of past illnesses or just of life well lived.

The scan found objects in Dr. Casarella's organs that are called "incidentalomas" by radiologists—minor tumors or growths, not connected to any symptom but clearly abnormalities that raise concerns. Dr. H. Gilbert Welch, in his book *Overdiagnosed*, explains that these kinds of abnormalities are extremely common, even more common now that we have CT scans that can see abnormalities as small as the tip of a ballpoint pen. However, he says that most incidentalomas are not cancer.

He writes that "with the exception of lung nodules in smokers, less than 1 percent of these incidentalomas could possibly represent lethal cancers. So more than 99 percent of the time there is nothing to fix."[5]

Most of us are carrying abnormalities in our bodies. If someone looks hard enough, with sufficient amounts of precisely guided radiation, they'll be able to pick up many of them on a scan. Then what?

Dr. Casarella describes what often happens: "The usual thing you do is to follow them [the abnormalities] with more CT scans to see if they grow—to see if they change their character." In his case, the lesions in his lungs looked suspicious so "the decision was made—well, let's just ... biopsy those and take them out."

He rather dryly told me, "It's a big deal if you have to do lung surgery." Since our lungs are shielded by a thick rack of skin, muscle, and fat, the surgeons had to slice through quite a bit of stuff to get at his ribs, and then they used a saw to open him up so they could get at his lungs.

Pieces of his lung were removed for further inspection. But these samples, like all the other things that had been discovered on what was supposed to be a virtual tour of his colon, were benign. None of the anomalies discovered by the original scan were ever going to hurt him. The months of anxiety, procedures, and surgeries were over for him.

Obviously, what happened with William Casarella had a good outcome. Everything that the virtual colonoscopy found was benign.

But what an ordeal. Was lung surgery actually necessary? Do we expect the medical system to dig deeper to see if all the suspicious things a CT scan turns up are trouble? Or do we discount the abnormalities, call them normal, and do nothing? Neither option seems satisfactory. Or maybe we recognize that incidentalomas are a normal part of scanning the lungs and we just keep an eye on them when they arise? Dr. Welch believes that we have to think about how all the high-tech scanning ultimately leaves the patient. He says, "I believe that if we could lower the intensity with which we react to incidentalomas, we'd do better by patients."[6]

Or we could rethink the way we apply screening tests for colon cancer. Dr. Casarella succinctly sums up his many medical adventures, the incredible anxiety, the near-death experiences of major surgery, the months of pain and recovery: "It was a lot of activity precipitated by a screening test."

AND DR. CASARELLA is not alone.

About 30 million Americans every year get a colon cancer screening test, but according to the Centers for Disease Control in the U.S., despite the availability of effective screening tests, colorectal cancer screening remains underused, and "lags far behind screening for breast and cervical cancers."[7]

There are a lot of unknowns about screening for colon cancer, even if it is one of the most scientifically justified types of screening. It is shunned by the general public. The U.S. government stresses that more than half the colorectal cancer deaths in the U.S. could be prevented by regular screening of everyone age 50 and over, yet there are things about the tests themselves that demand further scrutiny.

For one, most people should know that if there appears to be blood in your stool, you probably don't have cancer. The fecal occult blood test has "perhaps the highest false-positive rate of any screening test, between 8 and 16 percent."[8] There are quite a few other medical reasons why you might have blood in your stool that have nothing to do with cancer.

Then there are bigger unknowns, such as what to do about anomalies discovered during a colon examination. People as they age develop what are called adenomatous lesions in their colons. Sometimes they develop polyps, little hunks of flesh that hang around, and despite the fact these are very common, no one is exactly sure why they are there and what they will do. According to Dr. H. Gilbert Welch, about one in three adults has polyps.[9] Having polyps in your colon may not seem a good thing, and though they are not automatically considered cancerous, they have a potential to become cancerous. So we worry about them.

What isn't known—and this may be the most contentious issue around colon cancer screening—is how long it takes colon cancer to develop. Most of the recommendations regarding colon cancer screening use models based on assumptions about the "adenoma-carcinoma sequence"—how long it may take a simple benign lesion or polyp to develop into a full-blown cancer. Some say the average time is ten years; others say it's twenty-two years. Suffice to say, regardless of the model, there is an assumption that there will be "life years" gained in people screened regularly compared to those screened infrequently and those not screened at all.

According to the U.S. Preventive Services Task Force (USPSTF), there is convincing evidence that screening adults between 50 and 75 years old using any of the three recommended colon screening tests can reduce the risk of death from colorectal cancer. Because a colonoscopy can involve harms, and the virtual colonoscopy (Dr. Casarella's chosen screening test) can involve high numbers of false positives on the organs that sit around the colon, it's almost always better to start with the lower-tech screening tests. Doing so reduces the number of colonoscopies required and also reduces the likelihood that patients will be exposed to the attendant risks.

So when should people start being screened, how frequently should they be screened, and when should they stop? The ages 50 to 75 are not arbitrary, but are based on very carefully considered thinking and research into the likelihood of finding and saving lives with the various types of colon screening.

As of October 2008, the strongest recommendation (Grade A) from the experts at the USPSTF said that people between 50 and 75 years be screened periodically for colorectal cancer by fecal occult blood testing, sigmoidoscopy, or colonoscopy, adding that "the risks and benefits of these screening methods vary."

They also recommended against "routine screening for colorectal cancer in adults age 76 to 85," saying there may be considerations for individual patients and that they "recommend against screening for colorectal cancer in adults older than age 85."[10]

How effective are these tests? The trial that showed the biggest effect of colon cancer screening showed that the fecal occult blood test reduced deaths (tested over 13 years) from colorectal cancer by 33 percent.[11] The annual screening test reduced colorectal cancer deaths from 8.83 per thousand to 5.88 per thousand, or about 3 per thousand.

If the boosted survival rate was about 3 per thousand, you have to ask, at what cost? Were any patients harmed in the course of the testing? The majority of the patients in this study that had a positive fecal occult blood test went on to have a colonoscopy or a sigmoidoscopy. Sometimes the colonoscopy results in a perforation or other complications. When looking closely at the complications attributable to colonoscopy and grouping together the adverse events (including hospital admission, perforation, major bleeding, diverticulitis, severe abdominal pain, and cardiovascular events), we find they occur about 2.5 times per thousand.

What these numbers remind me of is that it's always worth researching—in advance of getting screened—what the numbers say about your likelihood of being helped versus being hurt.

What about the benefits of the more advanced colon screening such as fecal DNA screening or having what Dr. Casarella had, a virtual colonograph? The USPSTF recommendation (Grade D) said that "the evidence is insufficient to assess the benefits and harms of computed tomographic colonography and fecal DNA testing as screening modalities for colorectal cancer."

THE AMERICAN College of Radiology was effusive when it issued a news release of a new trial of CT colonography in September 2008.[12] The head of the trial, Dr. C. Daniel Johnson of the Mayo Clinic in Scottsdale, Arizona, said that "CT colonography could be adopted into the mainstream of clinical practice as a primary option for colorectal cancer screening."

The media was equally fulsome, saying that the long anticipated results of this trial meant that CT screening of the colon could become the standard screening method for colon cancer in otherwise healthy adults.

Yet the experts at the USPSTF had stated that it was too early to recommend CT colon screening, and that there were many concerns, especially regarding the finding of incidentalomas outside the colon, the risks of radiation exposure, and the fact that there is operator variability in interpreting the CT scans.

So why did the media jump all over these trial results as proof CT colonography had arrived? Gary Schwitzer has an answer. The former TV reporter and founder of HealthNewsReview. org leads an organization in the U.S. that evaluates medical news reporting. His group analyzed a story from the October 8, 2008, edition of the *Atlantic Journal-Constitution*[13] and gave the story one of the lowest ratings possible: a score of just one out of ten criteria deemed satisfactory. Their review called it a "very troubled story," akin to "cheerleading for virtual colonoscopy."

The media is vital in exposing consumers to the benefits of new technology, and marketers know this. Those wishing to expand new types of screening work closely with editors and reporters when they want to get the most favorable press possible on their technology.

The sins committed in that story are legion, including bias in the spokespeople quoted, citing only "fans of the approach" and not reflecting the evidence-based perspective of the USPSTF.[14]

One of the main issues with this story is one that Gary Schwitzer sees all the time in medical news reports: The story doesn't adequately describe the alternatives and exaggerates the novelty of technology. The story calls CT colonography "science fiction" and likens it to "*Star Wars*" and a "video game" language that might appeal to readers but does little to inform them of the value or drawbacks of the technology.

"Disease mongering" is what keeps stories like this alive: The prevalence or severity of a disease is exaggerated to provoke fear in the reader. Schwitzer's group wrote that this story on CT colonography "crosses the line into disease mongering in its description of a polyp calling it a "monster... sprouting inside a patient's large intestine like a mushroom."

The story suggests that most polyps develop into cancer in ten years. The reviewers noted that not only is this not true, but "this kind of misstatement does a disservice to the reader in obscuring the clinical reality with fear mongering."

We are a long way from the end of the story on colon cancer screening. The independent experts say it should be done, starting with occasional fecal occult blood testing, flexible sigmoidoscopy, or colonoscopy. If the goal is to reduce your chances of dying from colon cancer, the USPSTF benefit assessment can be summarized in two sentences: "Colonoscopy is a necessary step in any screening program that reduces mortality from colorectal cancer. This reduction in mortality does come at the expense of significant morbidity associated with colonoscopy."[15]

Like a lot of screening, the promoters say that colon screening should be done often and with the highest tech machines available, even though the evidence at the moment is inconclusive as to how likely it is that you'll be helped or hurt by such screening.

Perhaps it's worth reflecting on the words of Dr. William Casarella, whose own experience with the highest of the high tech in colon screening started him on an adventure he'd never planned on taking: "I think what I experienced and [what] was brought home to me personally was the downside of having screening and the false positives that had to be pursued."

OF ALL the medical screening programs offered to the population nowadays, which one gets the top spot in terms of potentially saving a person's life?

When asked that question, I immediately answer "the Pap smear." It's a test in which a sampling of cells taken from a woman's cervix (the organ connecting the uterus and vagina) are examined under a microscope for any signs of abnormality. While a Pap test is relatively easy to administer, many women find it invasive and unpleasant, even as it accomplishes what a good screening test should: It finds abnormalities in a relatively safe and efficient way, and early enough to be dealt with before they develop into real health problems.

Dr. Warren Bell, a family doctor in Salmon Arm, British Columbia, has performed probably thousands of Pap smears in his thirty years of practicing medicine. He sees the value in this kind of screening but has also seen how recommendations regarding the Pap test have undergone "boomerang-like" changes over the last three decades.

In the opinion of Dr. Bell, the recommendations for the Pap test shouldn't just be based on a random time interval, but should also consider a woman's socioeconomic circumstances, lifestyle, and sexual partners. To his patients who ask, "Do I need an annual Pap test?," Dr. Bell responds, "It depends."

According to Dr. Bell, "about two decades ago, the B.C. Cancer Agency, which reviews all slides from Pap tests throughout the province, made the bold recommendation that after a couple of initial normal Pap tests, and as long as your sexual partner did not change, Pap tests could be reduced to every 2 years. At age 35 or so, if the same conditions prevailed, they could be reduced to every 3 to 4 years. And after age 50 to 55, they could be reduced to every 5 years, and then ended completely after age 70."

He thought those changes reflected a bit of refreshing common sense, often missing in primary care. The principle behind the new recommendation was sound: Screen the population most likely to benefit and don't waste other people's time and energy. He thought that most women don't like getting a Pap smear and would've welcomed these changes. But Bell remembers that the announcement "was greeted with howls of protest from the gynecological community," which felt women would be hurt by such changes in policy. The agency hastily backtracked, withdrew its recommendation and went back to pumping the annual Pap test—another example where entrenched "expert opinion" slaps down common sense.

Changing recommendations around screening is almost always controversial, but when a change is based on new and better research and new knowledge, it's probably a good thing.

In the past, experts recommended women have a yearly Pap smear from the time of their "sexual debut" until old age, but how often do women really need it? That question is a subject of some debate, and Pap screening recommendations in Canada and the U.S. and around the world are all over the map.

In Canada, the provincial health systems in Newfoundland and Alberta recommend screening every year; other provinces recommend longer periods—every two or three years. The Canadian Society of Obstetricians and Gynecologists recommends screening every three years after a woman has had two normal tests.

The expert committee in the U.S., the USPSTF doesn't weigh into the frequency debate. It recommends "screening for cervical cancer in women who have been sexually active and have a cervix." For women older than age 65, the USPSTF recommends against screening for cervical cancer if they have had adequate recent screening with normal Pap smears and are not otherwise at high risk for cervical cancer. It recommends against it for women who have had a total hysterectomy for benign disease. The rationale here is that in older women, "the potential harms of screening are likely to exceed benefits." There's a final point (which may seem glib, but has much seriousness in it): Nuns generally don't need to be screened. According to the USPSTF, "there is little value in screening women who have never been sexually active."

Cervical cancer is usually slow growing and symptomless. It is almost always caused by the human papillomavirus (HPV), a virus usually transmitted sexually, of which there are many strains. In 2011, there were an estimated 12,710 new cases of cervical cancer in the United States and 4,290 deaths from it.[16]

Compared to other cancers, cervical cancer overall lethality puts it down the list. It is the twelfth most common cancer in women and the fourteenth most common cause of cancer death for women in the U.S. But it is the second most common cause of cancer death in the developing world, with a 50 percent mortality rate.[17]

One fact about cervical cancer seems stark: Not all women are at equal risk for cervical cancer. In North America, women aged 40 to 59, immigrants, aboriginals, and those from lower socioeconomic strata are all at higher than normal risk for cervical cancer. Most cervical cancer deaths happen among those screened infrequently or not at all.

Cervical cancer screening is a success story in reducing cervical cancer deaths. In the past fifty years, the developed world has seen a near 75 percent decrease in incidence and mortality from cervical cancer, largely due to cervical cancer screening programs.[18]

This point seems indisputable: The detection of cervical cancer in its earliest stages saves lives. Even though more than 90 percent of women will survive five years if the cancer hasn't yet spread, the survival rate drops to about 13 percent if it has. The USPSTF reports that if you introduce a screening program to a screening-naïve population (a group of people who have never had a screening program), you can reduce "cervical cancer rates by 60–90 percent within 3 years of implementation."[19]

More, not less, cervical-cancer screening is actually needed in the poorest parts of the world. This fact was recently reiterated in August 2011, when none other than former president George W. Bush announced the next phase of the Emergency Plan for AIDS Relief, which involves a major push to expand the screening and treatment of women with cervical cancer in the developing world, a laudable goal considering the worldwide burden of cervical cancer deaths—more than 85 percent of cases—are in developing countries.

Other than the Pap smear there have been other huge advances made in women's sexual health over the past thirty years, better education and protection from sexually-transmitted disease, and so on, but much of the success in the war on cervical cancer is attributed to the humble Pap smear.

Like any screening test, the Pap test can be overused, not only owing to the good income it can help provide for those who do the tests and the labs that analyze the samples, but also from patient demand.

Dr. Bell recalls the most overzealous Pap testing he's encountered: an 82-year-old woman who came to his office for her annual Pap smear. He said his "jaw hit the floor with a thud" after the woman told him she had had the test every year, all her adult life, and had never shown any abnormalities. She had also lived with the same partner for decades. Her reason for getting the test each year was simple: "I get it because I have always got it." He assured her she didn't need to have it anymore.

This same sort of overzealousness in doing cervical cancer tests in elderly women was evident in a recent report[20] by a U.S. group called the Center for Public Integrity. In a published examination of U.S. Medicare spending on such tests, they cited some truly astonishing, over-the-top uses of screening. Despite the era of fiscal restraint, the center found that U.S. Medicare spent "about $1.9 billion on common cancer screenings for people who were older than government-recommended age limits between 2003 and 2008."

By examining six years' worth of Medicare billing records, the center found that this "over the age limit" screening consumed "about 40% of everything that Medicare spent on breast, colon, prostate and cervical cancer screenings in that time period." The report goes on to say that "more than $31 million of that money was spent screening people who were in their 90s."

In terms of cervical cancer screenings, which the USPSTF says should probably stop at 65, the report noted that "over 80% of Medicare claims—more than 13 million—were for women who were 65 or older."

The report also found that many screening tests were being ordered for terminally ill patients, for whom the tests are idiotic and futile. This finding was similar to a 2010 study in the *Journal of the American Medical Association (JAMA)*,[21] which said, about 6 percent of terminally ill women covered by Medicare got Pap smears.

Of those with a "recent history of screening," 23 percent had had a Pap smear after being diagnosed with a terminal illness.

The chair of the USPSTF, Dr. Virginia Moyer, stated the obvious: "this is a very bad way to expend money that is in short supply" and noted that "there's human suffering involved."[22]

IF YOU are facing screening for either colon cancer or cervical cancer, it pays to do your research.

Start by looking at your individual circumstances, your age, and your personal level of risk. Look also at the independent evidence and recommendations for people in your circumstances: focus on the advice of independent experts like those serving on the USPSTF (Google USPSTF) or the Canadian Task Force on Preventive Health Care at www.CanadianTaskForce.ca/.

The lure of these screening tests might be more compelling if you are considered high risk (for example, if you have a family history of either of these diseases, or, in the case of cervical cancer, a higher than normal exposure to HPV virus).

Both cervical and colon cancer screening involve looking for warning signs, lesions, or polyps that suggest cancer. Once found, those anomalies often need to be investigated and tested further to get assurance that they won't become cancer. Screening might be appropriate, but go into things with your eyes wide open, and remember that most of the time your likelihood of having a false positive is greater than your chance of having a lethal cancer.

Forty years ago, the famous Dr. Julian Tudor Hart coined the term the "Inverse Care Law," which, in its elegant simplicity, states, "the availability of good medical care tends to vary inversely with the need for it in the population served."[23] The more urgent our medical needs are, the less likely they are to be met.

I propose the Inverse Screening Law is alive and well today. Much energy and money is spent on pushing useful screening tests beyond the need for them rather than focusing them on the populations who are probably at the highest risk and who would get the most benefit from them.

SEVEN

Mental health screening

We're crazy, just not that crazy

BRETT THOMBS has had a conversion of sorts. Thombs, who trained as a clinical psychologist and is a member of the Faculty of Medicine at McGill University in Montreal, recounts his early days in academia when he was looking at the prevalence of depression in society. He was studying how screening was being proposed by just about everybody in the field as a surefire way to identify people who might have mental illness so that they could receive appropriate care. When he looked more closely, however, he realized how all wrong it was.

His conversion came when he started closely examining the assumptions underlying the recommendations on depression screening. What disturbed him, he says, was that "the numbers simply didn't work out. It was clear that most people we screened didn't have depression."[1]

To check his conjecture, he decided to study how mental health screening was being applied not to a general patient population but to a "high risk" one: patients who had been through a difficult health event and who were assumed to be more prone to depression on account of it, such as patients in hospital following a heart attack.

What he found surprised him: Screening of all heart patients for depression was recommended without reservation by leaders in the field, including the American Heart Association, but it hadn't actually been put to the test. There were no clinical trials supporting what was a very "robust and aggressive push to screen all heart disease patients for depression." In fact, Thombs found that the recommendations pushing these people into mental health screening were much stronger than those for patients in general medical settings. This is important because health professionals in cardiovascular care settings typically aren't trained to manage mental health problems.

Thombs makes a vital distinction between screening otherwise healthy people for mental health problems versus assessing people who seem to have symptoms and want a diagnosis and a solution. He says that assessment to determine whether a patient has depression is imperative when a patient demonstrates any possible symptoms. The tests that follow help to diagnose and get to the heart of that person's problem. Going after otherwise healthy people who are not necessarily concerned about their mental health, he says, is a "whole different paradigm, because the patient isn't asking for anything. We're going to the patient and saying: 'You haven't thought of this but, by the way, it's good for you, and we're going to do this for you.'" He adds emphatically, "This is a whole different ethical responsibility."

He outlines an important theme shared by many critics of screening: "Before you go out and recommend a medical procedure to people, you have to have some evidence that it is going to have some benefit, you have to have some idea what it is going to cost, and you have to have some idea of what the potential harms are."

He says that supporters of mental health screening point to the growing number of people who are identified and put into treatment, either with drugs or nondrug therapies. Screening advocates look at those increasing numbers and declare success because more people are being treated.

But Brett Thombs says that isn't good enough. "If you increase the number of people who are getting a medical treatment but you don't improve their health, you are harming them." He adds, "Of the fifteen or twenty depression screening trials in general medical practices, some have increased the number of patients getting treated, but none have found that screened patients have improved mental health. Patients who are treated without benefit are exposed to drug side effects." As well, it sends the message "that they have a mental health disorder, even though they may not have thought they had a problem."

People can become confused about mental health screening, often praising the screening yet misinterpreting what it actually is. They point to studies that test whether people with depression who are treated or provided with collaborative depression care do better than people with depression who are not provided with that care. Screening, however, is not about treating people who we know to have a disorder, says Thombs. Rather, "it is about finding people who might have one, trying to get them into treatment, and hoping that treatment is successful. That is a different ball of wax, altogether."

But when you look at guidelines around the world strongly promoting the expansion of depression screening in the belief that those guidelines help steer mentally ill patients toward improvement, it's clear the belief outstrips the evidence. This problem is particularly evident in many programs designed to prevent teenage depression and suicide.

Most parents are confident that they'd be the first to know if their child was depressed or suicidal. Yet according to the Teen-Screen National Center for Mental Health Checkups at Columbia University, "80 per cent of mentally ill youth are not identified and do not receive services."

Could it really be so? These advocates and many others like them around the U.S. are pushing to get every American teenager screened for mental health problems, contending that "screening can help find those youth who are suffering from undiagnosed mental illness or are at risk for suicide." Screening will help in other ways, they contend, and can "make parents aware of their children's difficulties, and help connect them with mental health services that can save their [the children's] lives."[2]

Like all medical screening, this one sounds reasonable on the surface. After all, many teenagers are going through difficult adjustments, hormonal changes, peer pressures, and identity crises. We know that teen suicide and depression are prevalent. The U.S. Centers for Disease Control says that suicide is the third major cause of death in people aged 15 to 24 in the U.S.[3] If teenagers have undiagnosed and untreated mental health problems, and if we can do something to screen teenagers for mental illness— and help divert them from a path of destruction—why wouldn't we do it?

Unfortunately, mental health screening is a classic example of medical screening that sounds good in theory but is near disastrous in practice.

One need look no further than the example of the controversial TeenScreen program in the United States, probably the poster child for how *not* to go about mental health screening. Back in 2003, the New Freedom Commission on Mental Health, formed under President George W. Bush, recommended, among other things, mental health screenings for "consumers of all ages," including preschool children. The commission cited TeenScreen as a "model program."[4]

However, from early on, TeenScreen was accused of being a publicly sanctioned method of delivering millions of teenage children into the waiting arms of pharmaceutical marketers. One of the biggest targets for criticism of the commission was that the pharmaceutical industry was far too involved in its recommendations. One of those recommendations was that mental illness treatments follow a certain standard medication protocol such as the now infamous Texas Medication Algorithm Project (TMAP).[5]

If TMAP seemed like it was established by the pharmaceutical industry, it's because its policies were directly in line with the interests of the industry.[6] TMAP required, among other things, that physicians treat patients with the newest, most expensive brand-name antidepressants and antipsychotics rather than older, cheaper, and (some might say) "proven" drugs.

The adoption of TMAP was a boon for the pharmaceutical industry, causing the cost of psychotropic medication for Medicaid—the U.S. federal health-care program for people on low incomes—to increase sharply. The Lone Star State spent millions developing and promoting the guidelines, supported by funding that came partly from the Robert Wood Johnson Foundation, which has half its assets invested in the drug giant Johnson & Johnson.[7]

If you could get beyond the involvement of drug companies in designing guidelines shaping mental health screening programs, you might reasonably ask, Should we do it anyway?

There are certainly no easy answers and there are very good reasons for being ultra-cautious when trying to screen for and treat mental illness in teenagers.

One problem with the TeenScreen program is the TeenScreen test, and the vagueness of the questions. Asking vague questions to which anyone feeling even mildly blue might answer yes seems problematic. One of the more popular screening questionnaires[8] recommended by TeenScreen is the PHQ-9 Modified for Teens, which is described as a "13-item self-completion screening questionnaire designed to detect symptoms of depression and suicide risk in adolescents."

Given the ambiguity of the questions of the PHQ-9 Modified for Teens, its easy to imagine a teenager in the midst of a bad week giving answers that end up plunging the poor soul into the maw of the mental health system.

Some experts have acknowledged that screening for mental illness is only one part of the puzzle. They stress that screening to determine if someone is at "high risk" for suicide or depression is futile unless you follow up with appropriate, community-based help.

And although most medical systems are very efficient at handing out pharmaceuticals—drugs like Ativan, Paxil, or Seroquel to deal with anxiety, depression, and psychosis—they're a lot less efficient at providing counseling and community support to children at risk.

The advice coming from the USPSTF and its expert panel on teenage mental health screening said that screening was particularly helpful at identifying kids in trouble. Nonetheless, the panel recommended routine depression testing only occur if psychotherapy was available.[9]

In addition, using a screening tool to fast-track kids to antidepressants is a problem in itself. There is accumulating evidence, as well as federally mandated warnings, that widespread use of antidepressants in children may actually lead to an increase in suicides. Screening that results in appropriate care and actually heads off a kid who is thinking of suicide is a good thing, yet if screening does little but expand the use of antidepressants among the young, it can be like pouring kerosene on a fire.

Compared to the U.S., officials in Canada seem to have taken a much more cautious and slow approach to child mental health screening yet there are those that want to accelerate it. A few years ago, a Senate committee looked at mental health and addiction services in Canada and issued a report titled "Out of the Shadows at Last."[10] For pragmatic reasons, it was not strongly in favor of screening, citing the lack of appropriate staff to do follow-up and the impracticality of delivering a screening program across Canada's many differing provincial health systems.

Dr. Norman Hoffman, Director of the Student Mental Health Service at McGill University and a contributor to that report, said, "Screening programs such as depression screening may increase awareness of the problem of depression, but often all it does is support the idea that depression is a singular biological entity. This idea is highly promoted by the pharmaceutical industry, but has no support in the literature."[11]

Then there is the problem with the capacity of a system to deal with even more patients. The report acknowledged the constant challenge that teachers and guidance counselors face: having a proper strategy to help students with depression or suicidal thoughts. What good would it do to screen for more depressed students if we cannot deal adequately with the ones who already filter themselves through the system?

The authors say, "It seems unlikely that there would be a sufficient number of mental health professionals available in the near term to assist these children and youth. Given this situation, nothing would be accomplished by the screening; indeed, more harm could be done."[12]

Nonetheless, "Out of the Shadows at Last" underscores the idea that early intervention and treatment is vital for those who are living with mental health problems. The Senate Standing Committee on Social Affairs, Science and Technology said that the majority of mental illnesses that exist today began in childhood and adolescence, making it imperative to screen for childhood mental illnesses at their onset, even as early as infancy, and continue treatment where necessary, through the transition into school. [13]

Social worker Jo Ann Cook from Ontario would heartily disagree with that sentiment. In her work she travels between schools, holding meetings with school psychologists, principals, special education teachers, and others regarding students who are having academic or social problems. She is troubled that there has been a dramatic change in the way that problems in childhood are now being viewed. Teachers and other school personnel have been trained by "mental health experts" to be "disease spotters" (her phrase)[14] so that they can be involved in the early identification of mental illness and assist in helping students find effective treatment.

Many schools have been directed to take on this role of mental health screener, in addition to teaching. They have had to develop partnerships with hospitals and other community-based mental health services to assist them in identifying at-risk students.

As a result, millions of children and adolescents throughout Canada and the U.S. are being screened for mental disorders within the school setting in an effort to identify those with mental illnesses such as ADHD, anxiety, obsessive compulsive disorder, depression, and bipolar disorder.

Jo Anne Cook says, "The treatment is often strong psychotropic medications that can have adverse effects. The belief is that these mental disorders are biologically based, that medication can treat the symptoms and improve not only school performance but create positive child and adult outcomes.

"All children and youth are at risk of being screened and diagnosed with mental health disorders," says Cook. "Yet the most vulnerable children tend to be foster children, boys from single-parent families, poor and working-class children who have higher academic failure rates, and children who are experiencing some trauma at home or in the community." Cook also says that "there is no evidence that this group of children are sick, have diagnosable mental illnesses, or that medical treatments are effective in producing stated outcomes."

Still, one has to ask, What does hard evidence say about whether mental health screening programs actually work? The answer is, not much. The closest thing to a systematic review of the evidence of depression screening (or what they call "case finding" instruments) was done by the Cochrane Collaboration. Their review of twelve studies showed that screening—the type carried out by a doctor's office or in a general hospital—"has little or no impact on the recognition, management or outcome of depression."[15]

The USPSTF tends to agree that the evidence is paltry. It states that there is "insufficient evidence to recommend for or against screening children for major depressive disorder or MDD." But despite this lack of evidence, do they recommend screening of adolescents (12 to 18 years of age) for major depressive disorder

(MDD)? Yes, they do, but with a caveat: only "when systems are in place to ensure accurate diagnosis, psychotherapy (cognitive-behavioral or interpersonal), and follow-up."[16]

All signs indicate that screening is a major and growing part of many of the high-profile mental health public outreach initiatives across the U.S. and Canada. Undoubtedly, mental health problems around the world cause immense human suffering and misery, and there are few jurisdictions anywhere in the world where there are adequate support for and treatment of people with mental illness. But despite screening programs and all their attendant problems, one is left wondering if pouring resources into programs to identify even more people as mentally sick—instead of properly treating those already identified—would reduce the overall level of human misery.

This idea conforms to one of the central principles of screening: Don't screen unless you can do something for those patients discovered early that would produce an overall benefit to their lives. Otherwise, cease and desist.

Mental health screening is promoted by entities other than public agencies. There are online questionnaires: You can just fill out a few questions to determine whether you might be mildly, moderately, or seriously at risk for depression. One such online screening test is the Patient Health Questionnaire or PHQ-9 (found at the site of Mental Health America, one of the largest mental health advocacy organizations in the U.S.).[17]

When you read the fine print, you discover that "The screening test on this web site (PHQ-9) is copyrighted © 2005 Pfizer Inc. All rights reserved."

So here's a test that claims to be leading us to better health, identifying at-risk people so that they can consult their physicians, and it's created by the world's largest drug company.

You must always read the fine print on any self-screening test, and the fine print on this site reads as follows: *You should not take this as a diagnosis of any sort, or a recommendation for treatment. However, it would be advisable and likely beneficial for you to seek further diagnosis from a physician or trained mental health professional soon.*

HAS THERE ever been a period when you flew off the handle over little things? Needed less sleep? Felt irritable? Now ask yourself this: "Is it really depression or could it be bipolar disorder?" These questions are designed to suck you into the world represented by a four-page ad promoting AstraZeneca's drug Seroquel, the top-selling antipsychotic in the world. And what a crazy world it is.

A report from IMS Health on U.S. drug spending showed that the new generation of "atypical" antipsychotic drugs, including Abilify (aripiprazole), Zyprexa (olanzapine), Seroquel (quetiapine), and Risperdal (risperidone), is the fifth-biggest money-making class of pharmaceuticals in the world. Americans alone spend upwards of $16.1 billion per year on these drugs[18]—an amount that has grown dramatically in the last five years.

A few years ago, I noticed that the volume of antipsychotic prescriptions had started to rise exponentially and wondered what was fueling that increase. The published research shows that schizophrenia affects only approximately 1.5 percent of the population, yet how come treatments made for schizophrenia are among the most lucrative and widely used classes of drugs in the world?

One answer, in three words, is "bipolar spectrum disorder."

Classic bipolar disorder, sometimes called manic depression, is really a very serious, lifelong mental illness. It involves dramatic swings in mood that often last for days and weeks, oscillating between mania and depression. Yet its new variant, known as bipolar II, has snuck up on us and surpassed classic bipolar, with definitions having been widened to include people having at least one hypomanic and one major depressive episode. The depressive episodes are more frequent and intense than the manic ones, so it's often labeled bipolar depression and is considered part of the spectrum.

We all have ups and downs right? Many people experience strong mood swings. But if you're going to medicate people with very powerful drugs, you'd think there would be an equally strong effort made to separate the mood-swing patients from those with established bipolar. Experts can't agree on how prevalent bipolar disorder is. Some say it affects about 1 percent of the population, and others say it affects somewhere between 5 percent and 10 percent. Who is right?

It depends. Makers of antipsychotic drugs and the experts they fund certainly favor the larger number and the spectrum, by which they might gain up to 10 percent of the population as prospective customers. Drug giant AstraZeneca hit the goldmine in October 2008 when its antipsychotic Seroquel become the first medication approved by the FDA to treat both "depressive and manic episodes associated with bipolar."

To get some clarity on the topic, I consulted Dr. Joel Paris, a psychiatrist and professor at McGill University and the author of numerous books critical of the misuse of psychiatric drugs. His latest book, *The Bipolar Spectrum: Diagnosis or Fad?* is due out in 2012.

Dr. Paris has been openly critical of the expansion of bipolar disorder for some very good reasons, the most important one being that the proper trials of antipsychotics in "bipolar spectrum" patients have not been done.

As in any case relating to expanding disease definitions, there is the risk that a large number of people may face the dangers of the drugs and not achieve any benefit because they don't really have the disease the drug treats. Dr. Paris refuses to accept what has become a common perception among his colleagues: that "everything is a variant on bipolar disorder, where every mood swing is being interpreted as bipolar."[19]

A lot of the overzealous use of antipsychotics comes down to how mental health is screened and labeled. According to Dr. Paris, there are many variants to human mental health. However, as he notes, "Calling everything bipolar is just plain wrong: Calling a bird and a bat the same thing is just wrong."

Dr. Paris agreed that much of this inappropriate labeling is fueled by the pharmaceutical industry, but that's not the whole story. He says that pharma is just taking advantage of something that was already happening in psychiatry. "If the psychiatrists weren't already attuned to giving everyone a medication, the drug industry wouldn't be so successful," he says.

Another reason bipolar might be so widely diagnosed is because of the Mood Disorders Questionnaire (MDQ), the most widely studied screening questionnaire for bipolar disorder. How well does the MDQ work?

One study of more than 500 psychiatric outpatients found that the positive predictive value—the probability that the person is bipolar if they get a positive score on the test—was around 30 percent.[20] Another way to say this is that the test pinpoints those who actually have the condition only about one-third of the time. The test lists all kinds of bipolar symptoms, but it doesn't define them in terms of a time scale. This fact has been crucial in personality disorders being easily rebranded as part of the bipolar spectrum.

Let's say you have classic bipolar disorder. Do the drugs like Seroquel actually work? Dr. Paris admits the drugs do help some people, but that the old standby treatment is lithium, which has been in use since the 1970s.

In fact, in terms of drug safety, this newest generation of anti-psychotic drugs are among the most toxic, difficult to tolerate, and potentially damaging treatments on the market. Again, for people who are truly psychotic, schizophrenic, or bipolar, these newer generation drugs may help. But even for those people who are helped, there is an incredible cost in terms of exposure to the adverse effects, which can range from merely uncomfortable to life threatening.

Heading that list is tardive dyskinesia, a very common, serious, and sometimes irreversible adverse effect. Antipsychotic drugs can cause people to make strange involuntary movements of the lips, tongue, and sometimes the fingers, toes, and trunk. The person can become immobile and have difficulty chewing or swallowing. The drugs can cause diabetes and Parkinsonism, a condition in which people have difficulty speaking or swallowing, lose their balance, experience muscle spasms, weakness, or stiffness. Restless legs and the jitters are also very common.

People on antipsychotics are often listless, disinterested, and depressed, which frequently results in another prescription, maybe for an antidepressant. Despite an incredible range of widely recognized adverse effects, there are still experts who welcome expanded definitions of bipolar and more screening for it.

One such champion is Dr. Hagop Akiskal, a highly decorated and prominent psychiatrist at the University of California, San Diego. Unlike Dr. Paris, he happens to have close ties to pharmaceutical companies such as Abbott, AstraZeneca, Bristol-Myers Squibb, Eli Lilly, and GlaxoSmithKline[21] and would be considered a key opinion leader, the kind of doctor the companies love to have on the payroll.

This influential psychiatrist has written widely on expanding the boundaries of bipolar spectrum, believing it will ultimately benefit patients. This is a highly contested area of psychiatry. Other researchers like Dr. Paris say that when the boundaries are too wide, many patients are either misdiagnosed or overmedicated. He says that instead of widening boundaries, doctors should be cautious and conservative when it comes to applying the bipolar label.

For Dr. Paris, the worst part of the story is the marketing and use of these drugs in children. He says bipolar disorder doesn't exist in kids, but psychiatrists often treat the young as if it did.

"A moody, impulsive child becomes a moody, impulsive adult. They do not develop classical mania. That's why you have to use the term 'bipolar spectrum disorder' in order to justify treating them as a 'bipolar,'" he says. "And then they get the drugs." Last year in Canada, nearly 700,000 prescriptions for such antipsychotics were dispensed for kids under 13 years of age.

So back to the central question: Why were drugs like Seroquel—U.S. sales in 2009 were almost $5 billion—among the biggest revenue-generating drugs in the U.S.? Is it because experts are expanding the definitions of bipolar disorder, using screening tools that are accurate only about a third of the time, or because psychiatrists have few other options? Is it because these are among the most heavily marketed drugs to psychiatrists and because the loose screening criteria make them even more prescribed for everyone, even for conditions for which those drugs have not been tested?

What we see at the end of the day is a paradigm that seems to fit with the concerns about screening across the range of diseases. In our rush to do good, we are also harming people.

We can probably conclude that much of the population may be crazy, but not that crazy, even as we slowly learn that medicine's capacity for producing "collateral damage" is immense.

When we push mental health screening on teenagers and the end result is an antidepressant, we can actually increase the risk of suicide. When we take occasionally manic people, screen them, and label them as being in the bipolar spectrum, we are inviting them to swallow powerful and potentially toxic antipsychotic drugs. When we screen cardiac patients—without any proof that we are actually helping them—then add a label of "depressed" and a potentially inappropriate prescription to their list of problems, perhaps we're doing the opposite of what medicine strives for: first do no harm.

EIGHT

Self-screening for disease

Planting the seeds of self-doubt

ONE DAY as I was working on writing this book, I saw the email icon on my desktop light up. I took a break to check my email. I'm on a drug-policy listserv, and there was an interesting thread on it about ADHD. How apropos, I thought, so I took my attention away from one task (writing a book) to another (perusing a short article sent to me by a colleague). It was an article in the *British Medical Journal* about adult ADHD or attention deficit hyperactivity disorder.

The author, Scottish physician Dr. Des Spence, is refreshingly direct, saying the definition, screening practices, diagnosis, and treatment of this "condition" have been thoroughly corrupted by the pharmaceutical industry. "Adult ADHD has a drug industry flavour and a bitter aftertaste of bad medicine."[1]

Dr. Spence decries the profession's adoption of a "loose diagnostic narrative" around ADHD that "describes patients who are easily distracted, procrastinate, choose stimulating jobs, and are easily bored and impatient," and in a sideways comment, refers to online quizzes designed for consumers, which can "loosen the diagnostic criteria further." Then he let slip that he'd filled out a questionnaire on which he'd scored a "moderate ADHD" diagnosis."

This online test caught my curiosity, so I zapped off an email to him, asking which online screening tool was cited in his article. Ten minutes later, he sent back a link: psychcentral.com/quizzes/ adultaddquiz.htm.

I, too, thought it would be a good idea to do the test, which consisted of six questions that asked about such things as how often I procrastinate or if I had trouble remembering appointments.

This is how my results were reported to me: "Results of your Adult ADHD Quiz[2]: You scored a total of 18."

My results were accompanied by a message that said there was a good possibility that I might have ADHD. It went on to say that although the results of my test were not a diagnosis, I should consult a doctor or mental health professional—"soon."

I wondered, did the results of this test prove the existence of my attention deficit? Hmmm. Look at that bird outside my window. Maybe I should check my email ... Wow, there's my neighbor walking his dog ... Hope he doesn't crap on my lawn ... I think it's gonna rain ... Oh, right, back to the book. ADHD indeed. And a bad case of it.

This questionnaire is part of the Adult ADHD Self-Report Scale (ASRS-V I.I) Symptom Checklist. The checklist was created by some of the top experts in the field of ADHD, is approved by committees, and is found almost everywhere on the Internet. But is there a problem with taking an online self-screening test for ADHD? Can an online screening tool really help determine whether we have the disorder?

I decided to do an experiment on the adult ADHD self-test using my colleagues on the drug-policy listserv as my data. I sent the quiz out to the group, which consists mostly of Canadians and Americans, but also a handful of other consumer-advocates, drug-policy researchers, epidemiologists, physicians, and pharmacists from around the world.

Within two hours, my inbox had at least ten replies. Admittedly, it was probably a poor sample, as only the most attention-deficit disordered of my colleagues would have jumped to complete the quiz, eager to distract themselves from whatever they were doing. As it turned out, 90 percent of those who responded to me had, via the test, self-diagnosed as being moderate to severely attention-deficit disordered.

One of the people who self-scored about as high as I did on the quiz was Dr. Barbara Mintzes, an epidemiologist who works in the Department of Anesthesiology, Pharmacology and Therapeutics at the University of British Columbia. I have known Barbara Mintzes for about fifteen years and, as we'd worked together on a few research studies together in the past, I felt I could trust her insights. She has about twenty years' experience researching pharmaceutical marketing and has seen the whole panoply of marketing techniques.

When I asked her what she thought about her ADHD test score, she laughed. She admitted she did the test because, like most of us, she's easily distracted and the test was a good diversion from whatever she was supposed to be doing at the time.

"Seriously though," she said, "no matter what test it is, I always score as having the condition. I've done these tests with social anxiety, ADHD, or depression, you name it. I always seem to have it."[3]

I should add that Mintzes is probably one of the most well-adjusted people I know. She said, "These tests generally use broader, vague questions that go even further than diagnostic tools. Just about everyone comes out positive. The tests are designed to get people to suggest to their doctors that they might have a specific condition and to think of everyday experiences in a medical way. You see them on the websites of companies who have an interest in getting patients to see their doctors—to ask to be treated."

Mintzes went on to say, "There is also a problem that when people test themselves, they are never told the screening tool will actually have more false positives than real positives."

And that isn't so bad if, like me, you're just having some fun filling out an adult ADHD questionnaire with a few colleagues and discussing how you all scored so high. But this quiz led me to search for other online questionnaires, and I found one for bipolar disorder. The instructions said, "Use this questionnaire to help determine if you need to see a mental health professional for diagnosis and treatment of mania or manic-depression or bipolar disorder."

This screening test, the Goldberg Mania Questionnaire, was easy to fill out. It suggested that I'm very likely bipolar, putting me in the category of "moderate to severe mania." When I sent that questionnaire to the listserv, a number of colleagues wrote right back, somewhat elated, telling me, "Hey, I'm bipolar too!"

Now, I don't want to make light of people genuinely suffering from debilitating ADHD or bipolar disorder. But can a bunch of serious academics and consumer advocates so easily self-diagnose with mental health conditions through quizzes they find on the Internet?

Do I really have ADHD or bipolar? Probably not. But how can I be sure? I think those tests did what all such tests are cleverly designed to do: plant the seeds of self-doubt, a tiny idea that may, just may, put down roots.

This experience led me to consult Dr. David Healy. Dr. Healy is a psychiatrist working in the North Wales Department of Psychological Medicine of Cardiff University in Wales. He has probably done more to help us understand the influence of the pharmaceutical industry on the practice of psychiatry than almost anyone on the planet. Some have dubbed the Irish psychiatrist the enfant terrible of psychiatry, legendary for his close examination of data in drug company vaults that showed that antidepressants can cause suicidal tendencies.

His most recent book is *Mania: A Short History of Bipolar Disorder.* So when he came to Victoria last year, I sat down to ask him what he thought of the rating scales used to tease out levels of mental illness. His blunt response: "You need to be very wary of any measurement."[4]

Healy is aware that handy checklists are everywhere, sniffing that "the web has been a boon to screening." He laughs at the screening tools for "attention deficit disorder, which are reduced to four or five questions."

The consumer-oriented checklists, he says, are not just useless, but actually harmful, skewed toward false-positive results. "If you use rating scales, they'll often say 'you're bipolar,' or if you keep a daily mood chart—you have become 'mood disordered.'"

As someone who has extensively studied the history of modern psychopharmacology, Healy says that one of the biggest misuses of rating scales is how they are used in modern medical practice. In the 1980s, diagnoses used to involve professional discretion, but, says Healy, today, a number scored on a screening test tends to be seen as objective. He states, "Numbers create a problem that the drug becomes an answer to."

He continues, "For example, you might have an awful lot of symptoms of depression—sleepiness, low energy, and so on, and then you're told to fill up that scale. And as a patient, you're not told to exercise any discretion. Just tick the boxes, and you find you've become depressed. At least, you now have a score on the depression rating scale."

In his book on mania, he writes that the "majority of rating scales within the behaviour domain are simply checklists. Far from being information rich, they are information poor. The main advantage likely to accrue from their use is to ensure that a number of possibly irrelevant questions are checked off as asked."[5]

Why is this a problem? Healy answers succinctly: "The clinical gaze is captured by those whose interests are served by the measurement technology. Pharmaceutical companies understand this very well and now run symposia devoted entirely to introducing clinicians to rating scales that the company expects will lead to increased sales of their drugs."[6]

I asked Dr. Healy if this kind of reliance on rating scales is unique to psychopharmacology.

"No, I would say it's all of medicine. You used to go to the doctor. They used to have a thing to measure your temperature—they used to put a hand on your forehead. Then they checked your pulse, and so on, but there wasn't a hell of a lot else. You were meeting a person to talk about your problems. You went because you had a problem. Now the situation is, you go to the doctor with your son and the doctor and you are in the room with all the rating scales lying around. You end up with the problem. Increasingly you end up where it tells you, you have a problem ..."

One of the rating scales the modern doctor might have in his office if he sees patients like me (middle-aged males) is a checklist that might capture a number of my symptoms of aging. That checklist can help my doctor shape my symptoms into a coherent narrative that may spell one thing: testosterone deficiency syndrome.

You've heard of menopause affecting women of a certain age. Welcome to its pharmaceutically constructed male equivalent: andropause.

It used to be that slowing down, taking naps, and losing interest in sex were common for a guy approaching age 50, but if you're a pharmaceutical manufacturer keen on tapping the gargantuan market of aging male boomers, you find disease in the most mundane of places. Getting men to consider their flagging sex drive as a disease and then marketing testosterone to treat it has been a goldmine for drug manufacturers.

According to David Handelsman, writing in the *Medical Journal of Australia*, the last two decades has seen an "approximately 20-fold increase in testosterone prescribing, despite no proven new indications." While this is largely a U.S. phenomenon (but is also happening in Canada, Europe, and Australia), he believes it is being "fuelled by heavy direct-to-public drug advertising in the U.S."[7]

That sentiment is evident in the growing sales of testosterone products in the U.S., which in 2009 "rocketed 25% in the

SELF-SCREENING FOR DISEASE / 101

12 months ending in June, to just under $1 billion."[8] According to a Bloomberg Businessweek report, sales of testosterone products continue to climb despite the world's economic slowdown, even though "the recession has knocked the wind out of other 'lifestyle drugs' " such as drugs for erectile dysfunction.

On September 28, 2009, in one of the biggest drug acquisitions this decade, drug maker Abbott Laboratories bought Solvay Pharmaceuticals for an estimated $6.2 billion.[9] The biggest jewel in Solvay's crown was AndroGel, a top-selling testosterone product. One of the analysts watching the testosterone market said that there could be "double-digit growth for such products, figuring that only 10% of patients who have low testosterone are currently treated."[10]

How were the companies going to get that other 90 percent of men into their doctors' offices to get some testosterone replacement?

Through a self-screening test, of course.

In the summer of 2011, Barbara Mintzes had a very curious email forwarded to her from a physician-colleague at the University of British Columbia. It was from Abbott, the company that makes AndroGel, the testosterone supplement with the biggest share of the market in Canada. The letter explained that Abbott was starting an ad campaign and that soon doctors might be seeing patients who were curious about getting testosterone treatment. It included a copy of an ad that Abbott planned to run in a national newspaper, the *Globe and Mail*, during the next month.

Mintzes has a keen eye on medical advertising because she is one of the world's experts on the direct-to-consumer advertising (DTCA) of pharmaceuticals. She found the email (which had been sent to 60,000 or so Canadian doctors) curious because it referred to the 1.7 million men who might have a problem with a condition known as "low testosterone." Mintzes says that she knew that that statistic was a drug-industry artifact drawn from a "terribly flawed survey carried out by Solvay pharmaceuticals." The published article on this survey includes a disclaimer that the researchers used an arbitrary cutoff for testosterone levels, based on studies of much younger men. In this study, a man could be defined as having "low testosterone" without a single symptom.

A week or so later, she started seeing the self-screening ads in Canadian newspapers.

In the ad, which took up half a page, there's a granite barrier separating a man and a woman lying in bed. "Lack of Energy, Low Sex Drive" is etched into the barrier in big letters. It's a striking photo that sends a strong message: a marriage is on the rocks.

The woman is gazing at the man over the barrier; he's staring into space. The tagline tells it all: "Has He Lost That Loving Feeling?"

This ad was all part of a bold campaign to get men and their physicians to think differently about being male and getting old. It was part of what Dr. Mintzes calls an "integrated marketing campaign," because it included both marketing to doctors and the public.

Mintzes described the ad as "trying to show the wife looking concerned because her husband is not as interested in sex as he used to be." Mintzes found that since they were portraying a young-looking couple, the implicit message is that these testosterone problems typically happen to men in their forties—which is not, in fact, the case. It was misleading in other ways too. "Most problems with sex in marriages have to do with the quality of the relationship," she says. "But the ad was clearly sidestepping that likelihood and pointing in one direction: lack of testosterone. It suggests that lack of interest in sex can cause problems in a relationship, but not that problems in a relationship can lead to lack of interest in sex."

This "low-T" ad campaign is an excellent example of the corporate-sponsored renovation of a condition which has been called a number of things, including andropause (the male equivalent of menopause) and the more medical-sounding partial androgen deficiency in aging men (PADAM).

With this ad, the company was not marketing a drug but a self-diagnosis test. The goal of the striking graphics was to get men to go to the website www.lowT.ca and take the self-screening questionnaire, a ten-question "Low-T Quiz," that required yes or no answers. As is usual with online self-screening tests, the questions were broad and vague, asking if men found themselves falling asleep after dinner or feeling grumpy.

Many of us might regard the ad as a joke, but you would have to admire the audacity of the marketing campaign, in which the company didn't even name the product and also didn't state who was paying for the low-t quiz. (In fact, Abbott underwrote the low-T ad campaign and operates the low-T website.)

But it was pretty obvious to Barbara Mintzes, who has seen this kind of thing countless times in the past. Even though, technically speaking, advertising prescription drugs directly to consumers in not permitted in Canada, Mintzes has seen many instances of Health Canada not regulating drug ads that she thinks should have been banned outright. In this case, she was one of around twenty-five university professors, doctors, pharmacists, and other health professionals who sent a letter of complaint to Health Canada about this ad campaign, asking them to take regulatory action.

The "low-T" campaign was highly problematic for a number of reasons.

Most peri-boomer men my age (the age 45 to 64 cohort) would easily answer yes to at least three of the low-T quiz's ten questions, and, possibly convinced they have low-T, might ask the doctor for some testosterone. Although a conscientious doctor won't whip out the prescription pad right away because a male patient comes in with a low-T quiz, Abbott isn't banking on conscientious doctors. It needs to convince only some of the estimated 1.7 million Canadian male boomers (with a certain cluster of symptoms) that they might have low-T and hope that those men have the cojones to ask their doctors for some testosterone-based libido enhancement. But even if a man gets his testosterone tested and comes out with a low score, that is no guarantee that he has a problem. Testosterone levels go up and down all the time and many things can temporarily affect a man's testosterone levels.

Health Canada dismissed the complaint brought by Mintzes and her colleagues.

"They called it [the ad] a 'health seeking' message, and since the ad had no mention of AndroGel or the manufacturer, they deemed it to be OK," Mintzes says, still somewhat furious as to how they could allow this blatant example of "off-label promotion." AndroGel's labeled indication is for hypogonadism. Marketing it to "every middle-aged man who might have a low sex drive" is considered off label, because it's not the condition the drug has been approved to treat.

Barbara Mintzes says that hypogonadism, an uncommon condition that AndroGel is supposed to treat, is "usually caused by problems with development of the testicles at birth, or by radiation exposure because of cancer therapy, or it can be caused by problems with blood flow to the testicles due to surgery." And these patients might benefit from having their testosterone levels enhanced.

At the same time, she notes, "As a normal part of aging, men's testosterone levels gradually go down by about 1 percent per year, and there's a lot of normal variation around this range. This drug has not been tested as a treatment for getting older. It's been tested for serious testosterone deficiency."

Mintzes goes on to say that when you start testing every man who has some symptoms of low testosterone, "the likelihood of false positives—tests that would seem to show a problem when there isn't one—is also very high."

Are there many downsides to giving men testosterone when they don't need it? Of course. Testosterone tests costs money, as do doctor visits, and drug prescriptions can add up. Testosterone-replacement drugs can also have side effects, such as frequent or persistent erections, nausea, vomiting, or jaundice. And there is research evidence that testosterone supplements may increase the risk of heart disease and prostate cancer.

One of the weirdest things about testosterone gel is the possibility of virilization of the people you touch. If another person comes in contact with the product on your skin, it can seep into their skin, causing them to develop masculine traits. On this basis alone, the U.S. Food and Drug Administration (FDA) issued a "Black Box" warning—the sternest drug safety warning—that two types of testosterone gel caused the following symptoms in children: "inappropriate enlargement of the genitalia, premature development of pubic hair, advanced bone age, increased libido and aggressive behavior."[11]

Nonetheless, are campaigns like the "low-T" campaign effective in getting men to ask their doctors about testosterone supplements?

According to a survey a decade ago of 1,000 people, only about 50 percent of men said they would consult their doctor if they had signs of low testosterone. Clearly, there's a whole group of guys that need to be convinced they've got something medically wrong with them. Interestingly, only one-third of the women polled thought men would seek medical treatment for low-T.[12]

Self screening to drive markets for testosterone drugs, as well as markets for bipolar and ADHD drugs, will only continue to grow and thrive, if the public continues to be lured by the thrill of simple self-screening tests.

As the saying goes, the doctor who treats himself has an idiot for a patient. Maybe this truism should be extended to consumers who wish to screen themselves. They too may be dealing with a patient who doesn't see the whole picture.

Above all, be aware: A self-assessment test might seem cool and even fun, but before you take it, ask yourself if you want it planting, then watering and nurturing, that seed of self-doubt in your head.

NINE

Lung screening for cancer and COPD

Finding disease in every breath you take

WHEN A major clinical trial is halted, it's almost always front-page news, the equivalent of the Super Bowl in the medical world.

On November 4, 2010, the National Cancer Institute (NCI) in the United States announced it was halting the National Lung Screening Trial (NLST), an eight-year lung cancer screening trial. The NLST had studied 53,000 heavy smokers and former smokers in a high-quality clinical trial, comparing the effectiveness of scanning for lung cancer using CT scans versus using X-rays. Did CT scanning lead to the early detection of cancer? Did the use of CT scans to detect cancer result in fewer deaths?

The findings of the trial sent shock waves throughout the cancer-screening community. The NLST[1] found that using low-dose CT scans to screen people at high risk for lung cancer—mostly heavy smokers and former heavy smokers—"reduced lung cancer mortality by 20%."

The results of the NLST were important for a very good reason: Despite the fact that lung cancer screening using CT scanners had been heavily promoted to the public in the U.S., Canada, and other countries for at least a decade, there had been no high-quality research to support this kind of lung screening. Now there was.

This study was unique because it looked only at people from ages 55 to 74 who were considered very high risk, those with a smoking history of at least 30 "pack years." Thirty pack years means smoking on average a pack (20 cigarettes) a day for 30 years or the equivalent (for example, 2 packs a day for 15 years).

Although there were 53,000 people in the trial, the number of lung cancers discovered seemed small. So was the number of deaths. The trial had followed each subject for at least five years, and there were 354 lung cancer deaths in the CT scan group (roughly 1.4 percent of the total CT patients) and 442 in the chest X-rays group (roughly 1.7 percent of the X-rayed patients). The absolute difference between the two groups of 0.3 percent (1.7%-1.4%=0.3%) was translated as "20 percent reduction in mortality" due to the CT screening.

In other words, only 3 people in a thousand who were screened with CT were saved compared to those screened with the X-ray. The other 997 either fared the same or possibly worse.

Although a "20 percent reduction" might sound impressive, what it means in the real world is certainly open to debate. There are several disadvantages of annual CT scanning, including the radiation that accumulates with each additional scan, the potential for false positives, and the risks from all the diagnostic workup that follows a suspicious finding on your lung. In this study, the vast majority of findings that the screening discovered were false positives. Across the three rounds of screening, 96.4 percent of the positive results in the low-dose CT group and 94.5 percent of those in the X-ray group were false positives.[2]

I was struck with how few deaths there were in the NLST among the most high-risk people they could find. The average person on the street might assume the death rate for heavy smokers between 55 and 74 would be about 10 percent or even 20 percent. The rate in this trial, which followed those heavy smokers over five years, was less than 2 percent, regardless of whether they got X-rays or CT scans.

Why is it so low? The authors of the study note that this might be due to the "healthy volunteer" effect: People who volunteer to be in clinical trials might actually be healthier to start with and not representative of the general population. The true percentages in the general population might be higher.

Nonetheless, the skimpy results of the NLST were heralded as a breakthrough. The website ScreenForLungCancer.org captured the essence of the excitement surrounding the trial in a single provocative soundbite: *"Detecting lung cancer early can save your life."* Many groups supported the new set of guidelines that resulted from the trial, and the National Comprehensive Cancer Network (NCCN), a consortia of twenty-one cancer centers around the world, recommended CT screening.

But, really, how significant were the NLST results? Did they affect what the legendary U.S. Preventive Services Task Force (USPSTF) recommended regarding lung cancer screening?

Let's just say those results haven't yet moved these national prevention folks to change what they were saying about who should be screened for lung cancer and how that screening should be done. They said the "evidence is insufficient to recommend for or against screening asymptomatic persons"[3] with CT scans or X-rays. The USPSTF does, however, say that "No major professional organizations, including the USPSTF, currently recommend screening for lung cancer."

OUR LUNGS are important to us. If we don't breathe, we die. And the lungs can be a huge reservoir for disease, including asthma, obstructive pulmonary disease, and the most dreaded of all: lung cancer.

There's an extremely compelling reason why we might want to screen for lung cancer: It's a serious killer. More people die from lung cancer than any other type. In the United States in 2007 (the most recent year stats are available), about 203,000 people were diagnosed with lung cancer and about 158,000 died from it.[4] Most of the deaths were related to smoking, but not all. Of those lung cancer deaths, about 10 percent of the men and 20 percent of the women had never smoked.

If a cancerous tumor can be confined to the lung, about 50 percent of the victims are still alive in five years. But if the tumor metastasizes (moves to other parts of the body), the survival rate is about 2 percent. Lung cancer might be considered the classic type of disease that you want to find earlier rather than later, and this fact has led to the investment of hundreds of millions of dollars in research and large trials involving tens of thousands of patients.

One big problem is that there is no foolproof way to detect early lung cancers, even with fairly sophisticated imaging technology, such as X-rays, CT scans, and MRIs. These machines can help doctors only detect malignancies that have already been there for several years.

Nonetheless, there are many advocates of scanning for lung cancer, and a number of companies promote private screening. Mayfair Diagnostics is a large physician-owned company based in western Canada that promotes "the latest advances in Magnetic Resonance Imaging (MRI) and Computed Tomography (CT) technology" from offices in Calgary and Regina. It's one of many companies around the globe that offers preventive CT health assessment scans and screens for lung cancer, heart disease, and other conditions. It operates with a compelling slogan: "*When it comes to your health, knowledge is empowering and time is of the essence.*"[5]

They offer a lung scan for C$495, or you can buy the "Mayfair ASSURANCE" package for C$1,595, which combines both heart and lung scans with a virtual colonoscopy. Mayfair's claim about the lung scan is not as hyped as you might expect from a private clinic but it does reinforce the "test early" mantra: "After quitting smoking, early detection may be your best defense against lung cancer."

In a passing reference to the NLST, Mayfair states, "Researchers have recently demonstrated that routine CT screening reveals most lung cancers while they are potentially curable." And then they cite a study from Cornell University and emphasize that "early detection of lung cancers can mean a longer life and, in many cases, a cure."

Services such as those offered by Mayfair are popular among a specific type of client: large companies who pay for "executive health exams" for their CEOS and board members. CBC news reported in 2008 that these executive checkups are "commonly marketed as a yearly event to save time for busy executives."[6] It went on to say that this "heavily marketed but questionable service [is] offered by many of the most prestigious U.S. medical institutions, such as the Mayo Clinic and the Cleveland Clinic."[7] But is there anything wrong with providing peace of mind to those who want to lay out the cash to get this screening?

Executive physical examinations[8] (for which patients or their employers fork over a hefty fee for an extensive physical) typically involve a lot of screening. Researchers who have independently assessed these private screening mills are unimpressed with their services, calling them simply "bad medicine." One assessment, published in the *New England Journal of Medicine,* said such services fail badly on three counts: "efficacy, cost and equity."[9] The author, Dr. Brian Rank, called them "one of modern medicine's most expensive and least proven approaches to care."

Private lung cancer screening and executive health checkups may ostensibly be about trying to tackle and perhaps prevent disease, but are they the best way to go about reducing lung cancer deaths? Some experts argue that only by eliminating smoking and exposure to other respiratory hazards will we actually reduce those deaths and no amount of screening will make much difference.

There have been major advances in reducing smoking rates in most industrialized countries. These advances are largely not the results of health interventions or screening but rather of stronger public policies that ban smoking in public places, tax tobacco sales, prohibit tobacco sales to minors, limit tobacco advertising, and institute smoking cessation programs. Even so, many people still smoke and hundreds of thousands are still diagnosed with lung cancer each year.

PRIOR TO the results of the NLST, there was a lot of research on lung cancer screening in the U.S. that said screening was hugely helpful, especially in extending the survival times of those with the disease. That research was seen as flawed, largely because of the lack of comparison, or control groups. In addition, the issue of "survival times" is highly problematic when talking about screening.

In research, one must always be clear about what is actually being measured. In some cases, it is "survival" after a set number of years. The problem with using a ten-year survival rate as your benchmark is that if you diagnose people earlier, you can make the survival rate look a lot better even if the patients don't actually live longer. This phenomenon is called lead-time bias. But rather than measuring survival over a set number of years, it's better and more reliable to measure overall death rates.

Dr. Barnett Kramer, a well-known physician-researcher in cancer prevention in the U.S., has a sly wit. He has held some very high-profile positions, including as long-time editor-in-chief of the *Journal of the National Cancer Institute*. He is now the Director, Division of Cancer Prevention, at the U.S. National Institutes of Health.[10]

When I ask Dr. Kramer about lead-time bias, he makes an analogy, using the cartoon character, Snidely Whiplash (and, because I'm Canadian, the Mounted Police).

Dr. Kramer says, "I have a cartoon which shows Snidely Whiplash tying down his victim to the railroad tracks . . . Of course when the five o'clock train comes through . . . it's going to kill the victim. But if you develop an early diagnostic test, 'binoculars,' then the victim can make an earlier diagnosis of 'train.' But it won't change the instant of impact. And that is known medically as lead-time bias: that is, you may advance the date of diagnosis, but if you don't change the date of death, then any perceived benefit is actually an artifact. Since we start measuring survival from any cancer from the date of diagnosis, you can advance the survival rate with any early detection tool without changing the date of death. That is, you may advance the date of diagnosis without actually changing life expectancy."

So I asked him, if you push that analogy further, could you, with those screening tools (the binoculars), alert Dudley Do-Right to come to the rescue faster?

"That's the theoretical benefit. If you have an effective intervention. Then you might be able to change the ultimate outcome. But it's not always clear that a screening test can allow you to do this, so that's why we have to study any new screening test very carefully."

When the promoters of screening use survival rates to convince you of screening's benefits, they may be promulgating lead-time bias. Screening advocates often use the five-year or ten-year survival rate as a way to demonstrate the success of screening programs, but those statistics—as the Snidely Whiplash example shows—can be misleading.

Finding lung cancers early is not without its problems, and lung cancer screening is notorious for false alarms and patients getting needless biopsies. In the late 1990s, researchers were finding that CT scans discovered many more tumors than conventional X-rays but, because the CT scans are more sensitive, they also turned up many more false positives.

In Canada and the U.S., nonsmokers who have no symptoms are usually not screened for lung cancer, but the debate around whether smokers or even former smokers should be screened continues. Lung screening is certainly being marketed by private firms and those who offer executive health checkups. And some advocacy groups also promote it. But what do the independent experts say about whether even heavy smokers should be screened for lung cancer? They certainly don't agree with the promoters.

As mentioned earlier, the USPSTF concludes that the "the evidence is insufficient" to recommend for or against lung cancer screening. Its rationale was that because of the poor evidence on overall mortality, the high number of false positives, and the dangers of radiation exposure, it "could not determine the balance between the benefits and harms of screening for lung cancer."[11] In my opinion, that is why we need investment of public dollars in screening: so that independent experts can deliver a believable evaluation about whether lung screening is good for us.

Yet, after decades of study, tens of thousands of patients screened, hundreds of millions of dollars spent on developing an evidence base to prove that screening prevents deaths, the jury is still out on screening for lung cancers.

THERE'S ANOTHER lung disease that is prevalent and also linked to tobacco use: chronic obstructive pulmonary disease (COPD). It too has become the subject of an aggressive push to screen for its early detection. Patient groups advocating for COPD say that COPD is the fourth biggest killer on the planet and that millions of people don't even know they have COPD, which involves damaged airways and difficulty breathing.

The largest cause of COPD is tobacco use, though some people also get it from breathing in lung irritants over time. If there is an epidemic of COPD, it's because too many people smoke. All trends indicate that rates of smoking and even childhood asthma have been dropping for decades. However, the push to screen for COPD is fueled partly by the drug companies that stand to gain by expanding this market.

When you analyze the educational and marketing materials targeting doctors, there are two keywords that you see and hear everywhere, whether in medical journals, at physicians' educational events or in pharmaceutical advertising: *underdiagnosis* and *undertreatment*. These are among the most commonly used terms wielded by those wanting to influence and even shame our physicians.

This is somewhat understandable when you consider that shaping physicians' behavior is important if you have something to sell. Guilt motivates because it is easy to imagine the guilt doctors would feel if they were not finding and treating a patient's medical condition, like COPD.

An article in the *British Medical Journal* by Glasgow physician Dr. Des Spence describes a very good case study in the professional deployment of guilt and demonstrates how guilt is used to get doctors to start screening patients for COPD.[12]

Dr. Spence writes about seeing an email advertising a "high level" professional seminar on COPD for physicians. It featured members of the Department of Health and a "collection of baronesses, lords, professors, and members of parliament." The seminar had support and speakers from some of the major drug companies that manufacture drugs to treat COPD. Dr. Spence surmised the seminar was probably a thinly veiled politico-medico lobbying affair revolving around how physicians and public health authorities in the U.K. were dealing with (or not dealing with) the millions of people with undiagnosed COPD.

Many large drug companies, such as Pfizer and Boehringer Ingelheim, annually sell billions of dollars' worth of respiratory drugs, especially drugs for COPD. The companies' investors expect the executives to grow the market for their products, but therein lies the dilemma: How do you grow the market for drugs for lung disease when there is a limited and shrinking supply of smokers and people likely to get COPD?

One way is to bash doctors with the "underdiagnosed and undertreated" mallet, emphasizing that they need to be more proactive in recommending patients for screening. The other is to get younger and otherwise healthy people to start asking their doctors for COPD screenings.

Screening for COPD is performed using spirometry, a test in which you blow into a machine that calculates the amount of air the lungs can hold and the rate that air can be inhaled and exhaled. Your results are then compared with those of healthy individuals of similar gender, race, height, and age.

Sounds useful, but is this test for everybody? The answer depends on whom you ask. According to the USPSTF, "The benefits of screening individuals without symptoms of COPD are very small," and you would need to screen about 400 adults between ages 60 and 69 in order to identify "a single patient who may later develop COPD symptoms severe enough to require immediate medical care."[13] For younger people, you'd have to screen a vastly higher number.

The USPSTF also warns that spirometry can "substantially overdiagnose COPD in people over the age of 70 who have never smoked and can produce some false positives in younger adults."

Dr. Spence agrees. Despite the drive to diagnose and treat COPD, he wrote that "there is no evidence that screening people with mild disease will alter the progression of the disease." Yet in one study, as many as 35 percent of healthy elderly over the age of 70 who underwent a spirometry test received a label of "stage I COPD."[14]

These patients are likely to be counseled to quit smoking (always a good thing) but they are also likely to be offered respiratory drugs—perhaps an anticholinergic such as Atrovent (ipratropium bromide) or Spiriva (tiotropium). These drugs might be beneficial for those with serious COPD, but for those with "early COPD"? There's little evidence that giving drugs to those people will improve their outcomes. Side effects of the anticholinergics include difficulty urinating and dry mouth. The more rare and serious complications include heart attacks and sudden death.

Besides guilt-tripping doctors into offering spirometry tests, COPD drug makers know they need to raise public awareness of spirometry screening to encourage patients to ask for it.

One example of such a campaign is www.KnowCOPD.com. Billed as an "unbranded knowledge center for patients," this website is funded by Boehringer and Pfizer and a few COPD associations. The site features a classic five-question, self-administered quiz: the "COPD Population Screener™." It starts with the slogan: "24 million Americans may have COPD, but only half have been diagnosed with it."[15] You dutifully fill in your answers, print out the results, and give it to your doctor at your next visit. (For more on self-screening, see chapter 8.)

Your bedraggled physician, weary of being flogged with the "underdiagnosed and undertreated" COPD message, probably won't have any energy left to explain how a spirometry test is an utter waste of time for a healthy adult and he'll just give in and order the test. At least that's what the drugmakers hope will happen.

The world's major drug manufacturers, while trying to do good and raise the profile of important diseases, also pay for foisting massive guilt-trips on our doctors so that they order screening tests. The manufacturers also help out by paying for the testing equipment and giving it to doctors. The result? Tests will then be ordered, unnecessarily medicalizing and stigmatizing many people at low risk for a disease. And then many of those patients will end up on a drug that might not help them and could, in fact, harm them.

What a business "seeking sickness" is.

Whether we like it or not, many diseases are being subtly reconfigured as underserved epidemics. Dr. Spence says "underdiagnosis and undertreatment" drives the behavior of physicians in a way that is a "disfigurement and distortion of healthcare." He writes, "This is the theft of wellness."

I can't help but take a few deep breaths and heartily agree.

TEN

Bone screening

Selling screening

THE START of 2009 did not bode well for the drug company Merck. It was New Year's Day, but the mood wasn't festive because three published reports had emerged on Merck's best-selling osteoporosis drug, Fosamax. All three painted a particularly dire picture of the drug. One study, published in the *New England Journal of Medicine*[1] seemed to say that everything we thought about how drugs like Fosamax worked might be wrong.[2]

That study showed that women who took Fosamax showed increases in osteoclasts (a cell that destroys bone), even though the drug was supposed to make bones stronger by stopping the action of osteoclasts. Another study in the same journal[3] found that based on reports collected by the U.S. Food and Drug Administration (FDA), Fosamax might increase the risk of cancer of the esophagus. The last report, in the *Journal of the American Dental Association*[4] found that up to 4 percent of the dental patients at the University of Southern California who were taking Fosamax had developed osteonecrosis of the jaw, a destructive bone disease.

One thing was clear: for some women, the drugs weren't working as they were supposed to.

Lynne Bridges (not her real name) of Victoria, British Columbia, Canada, was prescribed Fosamax in the late 1990s, but she's glad she's not taking the drug anymore.

Bridges did not expect to be a patient. The healthy, 55-year-old publishing-house sales manager was walking home from work one day when she slipped and fell. She broke her wrist but, after a few weeks in a cast, was as good as new. Her doctor sent her for a bone-mineral density (BMD) test.

When Lynne's test came back, her doctor told her, "You've got holes in your bones." She was diagnosed as having osteoporosis and put on Fosamax, which was supposed to increase the density of her bones and prevent her from having future fractures.

Like many patients, Lynne took it for several years but found it inconvenient, so she got her doctor to prescribe a different drug, one that she could take only once a year by injection. It cost her C$800 per year, which was covered by her employer's drug plan.

After a second broken wrist, which happened while she was traveling in Cuba, her doctor sent her for a second bone density test. Her doctor says it showed "spinal bone weakness," and he told her to carry a backpack to strengthen her back, explaining that part of her treatment was weight lifting. While she wasn't great at following through on that advice, she did get in a fair bit of weight-bearing exercise, being an avid Flamenco dancer.

She's been living with the osteoporosis label now for more than a decade and worries about the drugs she's been told to take. She knows all drugs have side effects and was surprised to hear that the current drug she's taking can cause heart rhythm abnormalities.

"I'm not sure it's doing much," she says. She feels fine and wants to do more research, even though she isn't certain she really needs to be taking anything for her osteoporosis.

When Lynne was having these bone density tests (used both to screen for and diagnose osteoporosis), she felt she was doing what she needed to do to keep her bones strong. She had no idea that almost everything about the disease, how it is defined, and how it is treated is intensely debated and rife with controversy.

Osteoporosis (which literally means "porous bones") is an age-related condition that can increase a person's risk of having bone fractures. Many of the bone fractures that occur with age, such as fractures of the vertebrae, are asymptomatic (that is, you don't feel them), but others, such as hip fractures, can lead to hospitalization and sometimes death. In facing such a foe, physicians needed to find a way to screen people and identify those who were at higher risk for bone fractures. The goal, then, would be to prescribe a drug or other treatments that could reduce that risk.

Bone density scanning, or dual-emission X-ray absorptiometry (DXA or DEXA) uses low-dose X-ray energy to measure the bone-mineral density of bones. Lynne's story is probably played out thousands of times every day around the world, usually when women have broken a bone. And sometimes, when they visit their doctors, just worried about this disease called osteoporosis, they are sent for a screening test to determine if they have it. Of course, the main goal is to do something to prevent any future breaks.

The result of a bone density test is expressed as a "T-score," which is how your bone density compares to a healthy 30-year-old of the same sex and ethnicity. The T-score is very controversial in that it sets a cutoff that determines which women are classified as having osteoporosis (or the milder version, osteopenia). That cutoff is somewhat arbitrary and leads doctors to label those women with a low T-score as having a disease when, in most cases, the variations in their bone density are normal for their age.

From my perspective, after two decades of watching the growth of the osteoporosis "industry" (which some might call a pharmaceutical-industry creation based on a screening test of dubious validity), I always come back to the same question: When it comes to osteoporosis, is there anything that isn't debatable?

Dr. Ken Bassett is a medical-school professor at the University of British Columbia and has spent much of his medical career assessing the benefits of drugs and technologies. He had a front-row seat when most of the osteoporosis controversy began. And it began with a screening test.

In the mid-1990s Dr. Bassett was part of a team at the British Columbia Office of Health Technology Assessment (BCOHTA) in Vancouver, British Columbia. His team was tasked with gathering all the available evidence around bone-density testing and producing a report that would help advise the Ministry of Health about its appropriate use. Their report, "Bone Mineral Density Testing: Does the Evidence Support Its Selective Use in Well Women?"[5] was launched in 1997. At around the same time, a new class of drugs to treat osteoporosis, the bisphosphonates, was being introduced. The lead drug in that category, Fosamax (generic name, alendronate), made by drug giant Merck, was just taking off all around the world. Physicians were being introduced to bone-density machines, and patients were being told to go get their bones tested.

There was only one problem: There was little proof a bone-density screening program made any sense. In fact, Dr. Bassett and his colleagues concluded (after their exhaustive comb through the literature) that the research evidence didn't support "either whole population or selective bone-mineral density testing of well women at or near menopause as a means to predict future fractures."

In other words, there wasn't any scientific proof that the bone-density testing did what it was promoted as doing: identifying women at high risk for bone fracture so that their doctors could provide them with the education, counseling, and possibly drug treatment they needed to prevent future fractures.

It followed that if a person's bone density measurement cannot reliably predict who will go on to have a fracture, then testing and identifying millions of women as "high risk" for bone fracture was essentially a useless proposition.

You would have thought that intelligent heads would have looked at the data compiled by Dr. Bassett and his colleagues and then scrapped the entire bone-density testing industry. But that didn't happen. The enthusiasm for bone-density testing took off, oblivious to the naysayers and driven by a lucrative new drug market ready to cash in on all those women with low T-scores.

Sales of bisphosphonates grew rapidly. Merck's Fosamax had a fabulous year in 1996, its first full year on the market, generating $280 million in sales. Fosamax was soon joined by other copycat osteoporosis drugs, taking the fledgling bone-density drug market from almost nothing to nearly $6.0 billion in annual sales by 2006. This train hasn't stopped chugging either, and the osteoporosis drug market is forecast to reach $14 billion by 2014 as new drugs come on the market and existing drugs get makeovers.[6]

What Dr. Ken Bassett found incredible was that the medical community could accept such a narrow and somewhat arbitrarily constructed definition of a person's entire bone history.[7]

He witnessed the whole process of trying to prevent fractures in people become simplified and mechanized. He described the process this way: "You take a test, then you take a drug, and take a test again to measure if the drug 'works' and so on." Dr. Bassett said that it was somewhat absurd to think that this activity might be meaningful or reasonable. He stated, "I think it is really what we see as ... I would call marketization."

The problem, according to Dr. Bassett, is that bone health is complex, and believing that a single measure of a bone's density can accurately predict with any certainty what will happen many decades later is very wishful but misguided thinking.

The pharmaceutical industry knew very early that if it wanted to sell drugs, it needed to be involved in shaping the disease and defining the diagnosis, right from the start. It invested heavily to develop and promote bone density testing, using what Dr. Bassett has called "a disease-management model." It was a "very explicit strategy to manage women's bone health," he said, adding, "I think there's no doubt that it's a marketing strategy. It can be characterized otherwise, but in my own terminology, it is the best example of marketization, and I think it's the clearest and most successful one."

From the published evidence, the first major trial of alendronate (the generic name for Fosamax) funded by Merck showed that at best the drug might have helped about 1 percent of women avoid a hip fracture over four years. The company's clinical research also reported that about 1 percent of patients experienced esophageal injury as a result of taking the drug.

This randomized controlled trial, published in 1996 in the medical journal *The Lancet,* showed that compared to placebo, Fosamax reduced the risk of "... any clinical fracture" from about 18.2 percent to 13.6 percent, which meant an absolute reduction in risk of about 4.6 percent.[8] This number referred to any fracture (not just hip fracture), and most of those fractures would be the type of fractures of the vertebrae that happen as people age, which mostly can't be felt. So the 4.6 percent benefit translates into about a 1 in 22 chance that women would benefit from the drug.

What does Dr. Bassett think about the wisdom of giving these drugs to women who are otherwise healthy but have been screened by a machine and told they have "low" bone density? He says, "If you're giving them to healthy people, the burden of proof is so strongly on the part of the people promoting these products ... they have to be proven to at least do more good than harm before you can give them to a healthy population."

And twenty years later, as the evidence of the harms of osteoporosis drugs continues to accumulate, we're still waiting for the burden of proof on bone-density testing.

PRIOR TO September 29, 1995, when the U.S. FDA approved Fosamax for the treatment of osteoporosis, that disease was largely unknown to the general public or even to medicine.

To understand how we got from there to here is to understand the issue of surrogacy. Intermediate, or surrogate, markers (such as a person's blood pressure, body-mass index, cholesterol levels, intraocular pressure, or, in the case of osteoporosis, bone-mineral density readings), are markers for disease. Your high cholesterol or blood pressure may not be obvious to you, but you don't want to have a heart attack. In the case of osteoporosis, the reading of your T-score isn't as important as whether you fracture. Many women with low T-scores will never have a fracture in their lives, and many women with "normal" bone density will have fractures.

But the point is that a T-score can be measured, assigned a value, and a drug can be given to try to alter that measurement. The goal then, for those with a drug to sell, is to sell the testing first, because without the test you'd have no market.

A number of PR firms working in the field of osteoporosis in the mid-1990s were key in reconfiguring osteoporosis from a rare disease that was believed only to strike old ladies to something anyone of any age could get. And in the shadows, funding these activities were pharmaceutical companies like Merck, banking on a big market for its new drug Fosamax.

The strategy was simple: First, convince women at younger and younger ages that they needed to be screened for this bone-weakening disease, so they were urged through ads and so on to consult their doctors for a bone-density test. Second, the bone-density testing machines needed to be in physicians' offices, private clinics, and hospitals, so the manufacturers bought and distributed the machines. Third, the tests needed to be paid for, so the PR firms needed to lobby governments to cover the bone-density test.

What most people don't know is that if you define a disease broadly enough, you can capture a large part of the "healthy" population. Most also won't know that drug company executives found themselves at the table at a meeting of the World Health Organization in 1995, helping to create the very definition of osteoporosis. The definition they created was so broad—based on the arbitrary value of the T-score—that it meant that about 50 percent of post-menopausal women in the United States (or about 44 million women) had it. And the message that flowed from the popular press strongly suggested that even the healthiest people should be worried about falling and breaking a hip due to the weakening of their bones.

Screening healthy people is only justified on a population-wide level if the test is safe, accurate, and inexpensive and if the results would actually make a difference in a person's subsequent treatment. So how does bone-mineral density testing fare when examined with these considerations in mind?

If you consult independent experts around the world—those not selling mass bone screening programs or marketing osteo-porosis drugs—they generally agree with Dr. Ken Bassett's assessment from 1997: bone-mineral density testing is often inaccurate and can't predict with any validity who will go on to break a bone. And in the bigger picture of overall public health impact, the testing—and medicating of the test results—directs funds away from efforts that could significantly reduce the rate of hip fractures, such as promoting weight-bearing exercise, vita-min supplementation, antismoking campaigns, and reducing the intake of anti-anxiety pills.

There is probably no one who has followed the osteoporosis saga better than the New Zealander Gillian Sanson. Her book, *The Myth of Osteoporosis: What Every Woman Should Know About Creating Bone Health,* is a medical page-turner outlining the many miscon-ceptions and controversies that surround osteoporosis.

Sanson has seen how millions of women around the world have been frightened or coaxed into bone-density testing, given questionable diagnoses, and suffered the treatments that they are prescribed. She has written that if drugs like Fosamax "offered sig-nificant fracture prevention, it may be worthwhile debating the benefits and risks. But the majority of the millions who take these drugs do not stand to benefit AT ALL."[9]

She is concerned that many of the toxic components of the drugs stay in the body, and we are never sure what the long-term consequences of these drugs will be. Sadly, the safety record of bisphosphonates only grows worse with time, even as bone density screening programs deliver new batches of patients taking drugs. Fosamax has been on the market now for more than fifteen years. Even more serious adverse effects are starting to come to light, including abnormal heart rhythm; severe bone, joint, and muscle pain; and bone loss in the jaw (osteonecrosis). It has also been linked to inflammatory eye disease as well as cancer of the esophagus.

Perhaps the most troubling (and cruelly ironic) dangers are the bone-related adverse effects of Fosamax and the other bisphos-phonates drugs. There is evidence that long-term use of the drugs might actually increase one's risk of spontaneous thighbone fractures. Doubly ironic might be the recent Danish study on the long-term use of these drugs that showed they might actually *increase* the risk of hip fractures.[10]

Gillian Sanson reflects on the misguided model of treatment based on bone screening: "A diagnosis of osteoporosis on the basis of a bone-density test alone is flawed and close to meaningless. The widespread prescribing of bisphosphonates based on a bone-density diagnosis has the 'worried well' taking the drug in droves, believing they are preventing a disease they may never have."[11]

Nonetheless, screening for osteoporosis goes on. Even if you avoid the bone-density test, another potential danger lurks around the corner. A new online screening test called the "Fracture Risk Assessment Tool (FRAX)" is now being adopted by such groups as the U.S. National Osteoporosis Foundation. It calculates one's risk using age, gender, weight, and height, as well as other factors. Again, the question Dr. Ken Bassett and his team asked more than fifteen years ago remains: How accurate is the test in determining who will or will not go on to have a fracture?

In Gillian Sanson's words, the FRAX tool and the guidelines based on it are not very good. They have "drawn wide criticism from within the osteoporosis clinical community. Rather than excluding patients at low risk, they run the risk of casting an even wider net and diagnosing and treating much larger populations than those identified by a BMD diagnosis alone."

Like many disease advocacy groups, those working in the osteoporosis field recommend screening a much bigger population than is probably warranted. Even as the USPSTF recommends that bone density testing start at aged 65 for women, the National Osteoporosis Foundation recommends screening all women 50 years and older. Based on this, Gillian Sanson says that "it is estimated that at least 72% of U.S. white women aged 65 years and 93% of those aged 75 years would be recommended for drug treatment."[12]

In the hullabaloo over what to do about osteoporosis, we seem to forget the thinning of our bones happens naturally with age. For otherwise healthy women, your level of bone density is not relevant to your overall health. Women identified as having osteoporosis need not live in fear that they are walking time bombs.

Falls cause more than 95 percent of hip fractures. We know there are cheap and simple ways to prevent falls, such as fixing our sidewalks and making sure we use them to get some weight-bearing exercise through walking.

The question of whether you should get a bone-density test should be preceded by other questions: "Am I scared?" "Will the bone-density test reduce my fear?" "Will a label of 'osteoporosis' change how I live?" "Will a drug actually make things better or do I even want to risk taking a drug?" If you answered no to these questions, maybe it's better to leave well enough alone.

Despite the controversies around bone-density testing and osteoporosis, the U.S. Preventive Services Task Force (USPSTF) recommend that women 65 and older, as well as any woman with "increased risk factors that put them at risk equivalent to a 65 year old," should be screened. However, they can't recommend how often people should go for repeat screening or at what age people should stop screening. And the harm-versus-benefit profile of osteoporosis in men of any age is unknown.

Lynne Bridges has about ten years before she turns 65. Will she follow the USPSTF's recommendation to get a bone screening test? Probably not after what she's learned. She certainly wouldn't recommend women in their forties be screened for this disease. After what she's learned about the making of this disease, the screening tests and the drugs involved, she hopes people will share her awakening and "think twice about their condition."

ELEVEN

Gene screening

When marketing precedes science

IN MID-2011, an event of huge scientific importance occurred that shone an intense light on the future of medical screening, but it barely produced a blip in the media.

On June 15, 2011, the personal genetics company 23andMe announced that it had the DNA of more than 100,000 people in its database, which is probably the world's largest collection of individual genetic information.[1] This information was collected from paying customers, willing to give a sample of their saliva and as little as $99 in return for some insight into their risk for developing certain types of diseases or into their family ancestry.

This huge and growing database was newsworthy because a private company was amassing a body of genetic information so detailed that it might well determine the future of medical screening.

23andMe makes it very easy for people who are curious about their genetic past or future to get its product. The consumer just plunks down some money (it's currently $99 to get started with 23andMe), sends in a sample of saliva, and commits to a one-year agreement with 23andMe's Personal Genome Service®.

The pitch on 23andMe's website seems to offer everything but the kitchen sink. It reads, "Gain insight into your traits, from baldness to muscle performance. Discover risk factors for 97 diseases. Know your predicted response to drugs, from blood thinners to coffee. And uncover your ancestral origins."

One satisfied customer, a man named Kirk Citron, delivers a video testimonial,[2] in which he says he had a genetic screen done by 23andMe, and it found that he had an elevated risk of venous thromboembolism (blood clots). "Having that information, I believe, saved my life."

Those are compelling words for a service that costs a mere $99 and a spit sample. But there are questions that float immediately to mind: Is there anything wrong with handing over one's genetic information? How effective are personalized genetic services like 23andMe at trawling through one's genetic pool to discover one's risk of future disease?

The answer to that last question is, "Not very." In fact, after more than a decade's worth of promises from genomic cheerleaders, it's clear that genetic screening services have almost universally overpromised and underdelivered.

For one thing, the genetic variations known as single nucleotide polymorphisms (or "snips") that are found in your saliva may be "associated" with disease, but for most conditions there is no certainty as to what that association means. And will knowing the information provided by a snip analysis benefit or harm you?

One of the main problems is not the testing itself but the proclivity for humans to mistake association with causation. A test may discover a genetic anomaly that is associated with a higher than normal chance of developing Alzheimer's or type 2 diabetes, but that doesn't mean you will develop those conditions. And there's no guarantee that if you don't have the gene, you'll avoid them.

You often see peanuts and elephants together in the same place; say in a zoo, for example. Therefore, you might say peanuts are "associated" with elephants. You also often see fires and fire trucks in the same place. But saying gene X or gene Y causes disease Z might be like saying peanuts cause elephants or that fire trucks cause fires. Association is clearly not causation.

And what do you do with the information if you find out there is an association?

For example, how much do you change your life if you are told the average person has a 20 percent lifetime risk of developing type 2 diabetes, but based on your unique genetic code your risk is 30 percent? How can that be meaningful? Will you exercise more and more closely watch your weight because of this information? Maybe. Both nature and nurture are involved in determining whether any of us will develop a disease in the future, and being told you are at "higher risk" based on your genes may or may not help you.

Society's understanding of the interplay between nature and nurture is still in its infancy. Definitive answers obtained through personal genetic decoding are rare, but what isn't rare is the extent to which those decoding services have been overmarketed, often through misleading direct-to-consumer (DTC) advertising.

Helen Wallace of GeneWatch U.K., a research and public-interest group focusing on the environmental and social impacts of genetic science, has seen the marketing of genetic tests come and go for more than a decade. Ten years ago, she authored a study of DTC advertising of genetic tests and pointed to several prominent examples in which advertising hyped the need for genetic testing while misleading the consumer with inaccurate and hyperbolic slogans.

Have things improved in the last ten years? Not really. A recent European report said that "aggressive marketing strategies and slogans for DTC genetic testing might overstate the potential for predictive information of such tests and overrate its future health implications."[3]

Yet governments have generally stayed out of the way. There are no laws banning the DTC advertising of genetic tests in Canada or in the United States.

Strangely, one of the industries that did some early work on genetic research was the tobacco industry. They became interested in personal genetic research early on and provided some funding for its development. Helen Wallace wrote in a 2004 report[4] to the U.K. House of Commons that one of the side effects of genetic screening is that it helps keep alive an industry that depends on selling a product—tobacco—that we know is bad for us. If, through genetic testing, the tobacco companies could credibly claim that only a minority of people with "bad genes" need to stop smoking, then they could continue selling their product.[5]

The tobacco industry hasn't been the only group heavily involved in funding academic research into "genetic susceptibility" to diseases. The pharmaceutical industry has also been eyeing the genetic aspect of disease—known as pharmacogenetics—and investing hundreds of millions of dollars in trying to develop new drug therapies tailored to one's personal DNA profile.

Pharmacogenetics captured the public eye as far back as January 2001 when it, along with the move toward personalized medicine, made the cover of *Time* magazine with a headline reading: "Drugs of the Future: Amazing new medicines will be based on DNA. Find out how they will change your life."[6] Pharmacogenetics attracted a huge amount of hope, optimism, and public and private research dollars keen on using the secrets of the human genome to profitably solve the world's most vexing health problems.

Despite that early hype and hope, serious research into DNA-specific drug therapies has delivered surprisingly little in terms of treatments for the general population. Ironically the January 18, 2010, cover of *Time* magazine painted a more up-to-date picture with its lead story: "Why Your DNA Isn't Your Destiny." Nonetheless, the industry continues to attract billions of dollars in investment income trying to cash in on using your DNA to predict that density.

GeneWatch U.K.'s Helen Wallace, one of the world's most vocal critics of the modern push to use DNA to test for everything, reacted strongly a few years ago when a U.K. government committee suggested that all babies born in the U.K. should have their genome sequenced.

She says, "Genes are poor predictors of most illnesses, so most children would get misleading information about their genetic risk." She adds, "Most diseases in most people depend much more on social and environmental factors. Better school dinners are much more important for most children than genetic testing."[7]

The proposal that babies should have their DNA profile taken and stored at birth was ultimately rejected as being too costly, providing too little benefit, and being ethically contentious.

One of the main concerns about the services offered by companies such as 23andMe is the absence of follow-up. Most such services offer very little genetic counseling to help patients interpret the results and understand their risk. And patients who take their personal DNA profile to their own family doctors are unlikely to get meaningful help there either, as physicians are not yet trained to decode genetic tests. Above all, there seems to be no coherent way to ensure that people taking these tests know what they are getting into. Despite the promise of a genetic crystal ball, there is little chance that the patient who sent in his or her DNA sample did so with a reasonable level of informed consent.

THERE ARE, however, a few tests that can more accurately help determine a person's likelihood of developing certain diseases, such as a gene-specific breast cancer or Huntington's disease. But even then, genetic testing opens a whole new can of worms, replete with other problems and ethical issues.

Huntington's disease (H.D.) is named after Dr. George Huntington, who in 1872 first described this strongly hereditary disorder. According to the Huntington's Disease Society of America, Huntington's disease is one of the more common genetic disorders and afflicts more than 250,000 Americans who either "have H.D. or are 'at risk' of inheriting the disease from an affected parent."[8]

The Huntington's disease gene is dominant, which means that each child born to a parent with Huntington's disease has a 50-

50 chance of developing the disease. That puts it in a particular class when it comes to genetic determinism around disease.

Huntington's disease in its early stages often affects cognitive ability or mobility, and it can cause depression, mood swings, forgetfulness, clumsiness, involuntary twitching, and lack of coordination. Bev Heim-Myers, the CEO of the Huntington Society of Canada told me, "It's like having Alzheimer's, Parkinson's or ALS and schizophrenia, all in one disease. It's emotional trauma and behavioral instability. It's cognitive decline and physical decline."[9] Eventually the person dies from complications such as choking, infection, or heart failure.

There are currently no treatments that will slow down or stop the disease. Huntington's societies around the world focus primarily on advocacy and support of people with the disease, and they have been front and center on the debates around genetic discrimination.

Heim-Myers would be the first to admit that getting any kind of screening test for a disease could substantially alter your life in ways that are entirely unexpected. It can leave people with dilemmas they've never considered before, and it often produces more questions than answers. She notes that many people who agree to be screened have no idea of the downside to testing. She says, "People go into it with curiosity and come out distraught."

Worse yet, it may set you up for discrimination. The United States and other developed countries have legislation that protects people from genetic discrimination, but Canada does not. And of course, you only know if you've got the gene if you agree to be screened for it.

That poses practical dilemmas, says Heim-Myers. She states, "If you are from a Huntington family, the insurance companies won't cover you." In fact, "there are many examples of people with Huntington's disease who could not get life insurance or disability insurance because of their family history."

This sense of serious discrimination is backed up by research. A published Canadian survey found that nearly 40 percent of respondents "at risk" of Huntington's reported discrimination because of family history or genetic test results. The survey noted that it wasn't the genetic testing itself that caused people to experience some sort of genetic discrimination—it was just having a family history of Huntington's disease that made many people feel they were experiencing genetic discrimination.[10]

So what do you do if there is confirmed Huntington's disease in your family tree? Do you get screened for it? Do you even tell anyone? While most Huntington groups would recommend the test for people with a family history of the disease, the bottom line for Heim-Myers is that "people need to make an informed choice."

There's that medical screening refrain again: "Informed choice."

Heim-Meyers says informed choice is about looking at how the test can serve you.

Learning early that there is a strong likelihood that you've got a disease like Huntington's in your family might allow you more time to prepare yourself for what will inevitably come. It also might help you decide whether you'd rather adopt children than risk passing on the Huntington gene. Either way, it's obvious that jumping into a screening test to determine if you have the Huntington gene is not an easy decision. As with any form of screening, once you've been tested you can't unknow what you know. Will the test change your life? Probably it will, in some unforeseen way. Will that change be only positive? The jury is still out on that one.

Some would argue that a personalized genetic test not only allows you glimpses into the depths of your own genetic makeup, but also provides an altruistic way for you to contribute your DNA to a worthy cause. Some day human DNA databases like 23andMe might be hundreds of times more powerful than they currently are, helping to lead to genetic discoveries that may allow more of us to live better and longer lives. That's the hope. But we're far from there today, and most online genetic screening and searching is little more than an amusing genetic horoscope.

"THIS WILL only hurt a little," says the nurse as she cradles a brand new baby girl, all glowing pink. "We're just going to take a little blood from her heel," she adds, as she swabs the tiny foot, no bigger than the nurse's thumb.

With one poke, a few droplets of blood are squeezed onto a filter paper and the baby's brief, high-decibel howl signals the nurse's job is done. The blood spot card dries and is quickly whisked off to the lab for analysis.

The nurse assures the new parents, a bit bemused and exhausted from the birth ordeal, the heel-prick test is necessary to find certain congenital disorders they should know about right away. Other than testing that little spot of blood for PKU (a genetic disorder that causes mental illness if left untreated) and congenital hypothyroidism (a disorder of the thyroid gland), both of which are worth finding out about sooner rather than later, how many tests will that little blood spot go through?

It depends on where you live.

According to Perinatal Services B.C., the group that runs newborn screening in the province of British Columbia, Canada, the blood of all babies born in British Columbia is tested for twenty-two different diseases. In the United States, the number of tests varies state by state, with some jurisdictions screening the blood for as many as one hundred different conditions.

All that screening seems reasonable only if something can be done about any disease that's detected. If the test detects markers for cystic fibrosis, sickle cell disease, or other treatable disorders, meaning that the child will need special treatment in order to avoid developmental disorders, liver problems, or brain damage, then these tests might be worth doing. But is there any downside to testing so early in our cradle-to-grave medical screening culture?

There's the cost, for one thing. It might seem to be inexpensive to spend about C$100 per screened child to find these extremely rare diseases, but cumulatively, it adds up. British Columbia's newborn screening program costs several million dollars to collect and test blood samples from about 45,000 babies born in the province every year. The tests will detect one of a handful of treatable conditions in roughly 20 of those babies. Another 20 might test positive for a rare disease, and knowing this information may be of some use.

When you do the math, you're finding some disease in about 40 kids a year out of 45,000 tested. That means for every 1,100 babies screened, you might find one with an abnormality you can do something about.

However, in some jurisdictions, they might be screening for diseases at childbirth that aren't so easily treatable. It is also possible the test might miss something important or find something that turns out to be insignificant. Then there is the problem of privacy and confidentiality. Can we be confident that whoever has control over a baby's genetic sample won't make it available to insurers, health authorities, or even the police sometime in the future?

Regardless of the best intentions of our medical authorities, we can't ignore the powerful commercial interests swirling around the decoding of the human genome and the fact that companies will pay handsomely for the kind of data generated by a databank containing the DNA sequences of all of our children.

Health authorities around the world are tasked with an incredibly important job: ensuring babies' blood samples are collected in the most ethical way (which usually means through fully informed consent) and guarded by the strongest protection possible. But how does it work out in the real world? This controversy erupted in Britain in late 2011 when it was revealed that hospitals in the U.K. were storing babies' blood samples for indefinite periods of time.

One of the U.K.'s major daily papers, the *Telegraph*, reported that "blood samples taken in heel-prick tests to screen for serious conditions are being held for years by some hospitals and can be subsequently accessed by the police to identify people involved in crimes."[11]

This concerned Helen Wallace of GeneWatch U.K., who said, "We do not want to put mothers off having these tests as they are very important for their babies' health, but the key issue really is how long these samples are being stored for." Like many critics worried about what happens with genetic information, she would like those samples destroyed after a certain period of time.

This seems to be an issue across other jurisdictions. A lawsuit brought against the Provincial Health Services Authority (PHSA) in British Columbia, Canada, on behalf of a parent charged that the government of British Columbia has been collecting and storing newborn blood samples from both British Columbia and the Yukon without the consent of parents. Jason Gratl, the Vancouver lawyer arguing the case, said that the government of British Columbia "has a secret and long-term DNA storage bank that was obtained unlawfully." He says this DNA information "can say a lot about the children who donated the blood, but it could also say something about their parents." It appears the samples are being used in research, but, Gratl says, "the precise conditions under which the samples are being used for research have yet to be explored."[12]

The tests for PKU and hyperthyroidism are generally accepted because the tests are accurate and early intervention will help treat the children with these conditions. But what about the range of DNA tests that could be performed on a newborn's blood? Is it wise to be testing just because we can?

The most sensible answer seems to be "It depends." It depends how health authorities intend to use a baby's DNA. Will they eventually attach that DNA to the child's electronic health record, fusing personal genetic and health information so that research and monitoring of disease can be done more efficiently? In some eyes, that scenario might be ideal. Others take a more jaundiced view of how that information will be used.

According to GeneWatch U.K.'s Helen Wallace, much of activity around collecting and storing DNA is already a boondoggle. She wrote that "billions in taxpayers' money has been wasted in both Britain and the USA and medical privacy has been jeopardized, in an attempt to create the vast databases of electronic medical records linked to DNA that will supposedly allow scientists to 'predict and prevent' disease."[13] In her opinion, "a massive expansion in the drug market is predicted if everyone is tested."

What is clear to me—perhaps best symbolized by this ritualistic bloodletting of a day-old infant—is that genetics is going mainstream and playing an increasingly larger role in medical screening and the provision of health care. The heel-prick hurts the baby temporarily, yet her first outside-the-womb screening test will surely not be her last. With modern health-care systems driven to screen for any and all diseases, this baby will face a lifetime of attempts to find disease in her body.

Right now, parents hand over their infant's DNA because it appears that the benefits exceed the risks. The problem is that we are not clear what we are risking. Will that little girl have a black cloud of a disease (which might never develop) hanging over her head or a greater lifetime risk of depression or anxiety? Or will she be discriminated against or stigmatized? Those are things we can't yet answer. Genetic screening of our babies may allow us to know many things even as it undermines something many of us hold as sacred: the right, sometimes, not to know.

THERE IS one other area where genetic testing is in a race to find diseases in people, and that is at the other end of life's journey: dementia. A perfect storm consisting of an aging population and the demand for future potential Alzheimer's treatments is driving genetic research to determine markers that can predict the onset of dementia. In this case, again, the promotion and the marketing precedes the science by many years, often engendering false hope and unrealistic expectations.

It's pretty clear that the groups that work on advocacy and support for Alzheimer's patients express a powerful need to screen. Alzheimer's Disease International, a London-based consumer group, says 35.6 million people worldwide are living with dementia.[14]

A major thrust of Alzheimer's Disease International[15] is early diagnosis, and the title of their World Alzheimer's Report 2011 is "The Benefits of Early Diagnosis and Intervention."[16] The authors state, "We have identified that lack of detection is a significant barrier to improving lives of people with Alzheimer's disease and other dementias, their families and carers."[17]

Although the seventy-two-page report emphasizes on almost every page the need to carry out and support the early diagnosis of Alzheimer's disease, buried in the report is a frank admission that there is no substantive research that doing so would make any difference. The authors wrote, "We found a surprising lack of research conducted into the effect of the timing of dementia diagnosis upon subsequent disease course and outcomes for the person with dementia and their carers."[18]

But why let evidence get in the way? The report's authors sidestep this issue and say that despite the lack of research evidence on dementia screening "it is clear that informed and expert opinion is generally of the view that early dementia diagnosis is beneficial to patients, carers, and society and should therefore be promoted."[19]

We know that early diagnosis is like a feedbag to the pharmaceutical industry, and the earlier the better. Better yet if markers could be discovered for Alzheimer's in a person's twenties, thirties, or forties so that person could become a lifelong patient for preventive treatments. It is important to recognize that many if not most of the Alzheimer's associations around the world get partial funding and donations from the pharmaceutical industry, especially those companies that make Alzheimer's treatments.

Despite a potential pharma-funded drive toward early diagnosis, and the dominant public discourse that says the aging of the population represents a worldwide tsunami of dementia coming our way, we know almost nothing about what causes dementia, how to prevent it, or how to treat it. Researchers in the U.S. recently analyzed twenty-five systematic reviews and 250 primary research studies in an attempt to determine the factors that cause Alzheimer's or cognitive decline.[20] They did not find definitive causes.

They found that diabetes, a certain kind of gene (APOE-E4), depression, and smoking were associated with an increased risk of developing Alzheimer's. Peanuts and elephants were seen in the same room. Factors that decreased one's risk for future dementia included keeping mentally and physically active, though the quality of the research evidence on this is poor.

Nonetheless, Alzheimer's disease is increasingly a target for genetic analysis.

There are currently four gene mutations that are related to the development of Alzheimer's, three of which probably account for fewer than 1 percent of all cases. The one of most interest is the gene that encodes the production of a protein called apolipoprotein E, (APOE-E4). It is linked to an increased risk of developing late-onset Alzheimer's (the type that typically strikes after age 55). While APOE-E4 might mean you have a greater risk of getting Alzheimer's than average, it doesn't mean you will definitely develop the disease. In fact, some people inheriting APOE-E4 from both parents never get the disease, and others who develop Alzheimer's do not have any APOE-E4 genes.

The one big elephant in the room here is a question that springs from the race to find a better test to predict who will develop Alzheimer's: What are we going to do with that information? If, in fact, detecting Alzheimer's disease early is based on the possibility of altering the course of the disease, and there is no therapy proven to slow or alter the course of Alzheimer's, one really must ask, "Why test any healthy people for Alzheimer's in the first place?"

The Alzheimer Society of Canada (which also accepts funding from the pharmaceutical industry) says that dementia-related issues, such as "motor vehicle accidents, medication errors, and financial difficulties," could be avoided by earlier diagnoses of the disease. It professes that finding Alzheimer's early will help individuals have more time "to adjust to the diagnosis."[21]

Although that sounds plausible, it seems that testing people for Alzheimer's—possibly applying a "pre-Alzheimer's" label ten or twenty or thirty years before a person develops any symptoms—without having something substantial to give them is like applying a cruel death sentence with no date as to when it will happen.

The energetic search to determine the risk for Alzheimer's before it strikes has fostered whole industries of scientists looking for biomarkers (or biological signals) that they hope will show if a person is at risk of the disease before any symptoms manifest. Finding these "risk factors" involves some very invasive tests, including CT scans of the brain (to identify changes in brain structure) and spinal taps (to identify protein fragments that may be linked to Alzheimer's disease). So far, these tests haven't been definitive and they have failed to pass the first few hurdles of an acceptable screening test. They are not simple, absolutely safe, or very reliable.

Part of this push is based on scientists' need to rewrite the definition of Alzheimer's. They argue that it should be classified as a "clinical-biological syndrome." One way to establish a diagnosis would be to base it not only on symptoms of dementia (forgetfulness, confusion and so on) but also on "biomarkers" such as a protein called beta-amyloid found in the fluid of the spinal cord that is "associated" with the type of plaques linked to Alzheimer's. But if a person is already exhibiting mild signs of cognitive impairment, why go to the trouble to define Alzheimer's in terms of a biomarker, you might ask?

Because that's where the money is.

If you've got a biomarker, you can develop a drug (as companies such as Pfizer and Eli Lilly are trying to do) to work against the biomarker. On that front, things aren't going as well as planned for the drug companies. Just recently, the drug giant Eli Lilly halted two clinical trials when two of its Alzheimer's drugs in development (which were supposed to reduce plaque in the brain) made people more cognitively impaired and less able to look after themselves than those on placebo.[22]

So should we be putting so much effort into trying to find pre-Alzheimer's and somehow stop it in its tracks if we can?

Alzheimer's is certainly a dreadful disease, and most of us would choose to avoid it at almost any cost. As you lose mental function, your brain cells deteriorate and you become more confused and disoriented. You stop recognizing people you've known and loved all your life. It's terrible. But would being screened and finding out that you might get it make it somewhere down the road any less terrible?

At the same time, the drive to screen people for Alzheimer's doesn't seem to be seriously questioned in the medical community because most people believe strongly in the "test early, test often" paradigm. That paradigm has been shown to have serious flaws when studied intensely (as it has been with mammography and prostate cancer screening), so the question we should be asking is "Why should we expect anything different with Alzheimer's?"

Will genetic discoveries someday help humanity by offering valid screening tests that can help us predict future risks of disease such as dementia? Maybe it will, and we can hope that research will continue to push the boundaries of human knowledge in this direction. At the same time, we have to remain skeptical of the hype around the human genome and ask some hard questions when someone wants some of our saliva, a bit of our baby's blood, or a spinal tap and in return offers us a genetic crystal ball.

A conversation starter when facing screening

What happens if I do nothing?

MY FRIEND Wendy Armstrong, was the first person I called when, many years ago now, I saw that flyer that read, "A Full Body Scan Can Save Your Life."

"We need to study this," I told her.

"You bet we do," she said.

As a former nurse and a consumer advocate for over two decades with the Alberta Chapter of the Consumers' Association of Canada, Wendy has deeper insights than anyone on the prickly subject of human interactions with the medical system. She intuitively understands human concerns around sickness and medical care, the faith we place in systems and health-care professionals, and the powerful longing that many of us have to do whatever is needed to prevent illness. And she also understands why people want to "do something," even if it might not be in their best interests.

Wendy likes to put me in my place, and we often debate, which is frequently fun and illuminating. Well, it is for me.

For example, she thinks I'm too obsessed with numbers. As a researcher working with epidemiologists, I usually try to find out how sensible something might be by looking at quantitative data. For me, that's the starting gate. Has this thing—whether it's a procedure, a drug, or a screening program—even been tested? How has it been tested? Do we trust those tests? What do the numbers say? And perhaps most important to me: Why does the evidence get so twisted along the path to the consumer?

Yeah, she says, all that's important. But she argues for a deeper analysis of screening: "There is a need to understand and speak to the context and underlying psychology and heuristics at play," she says, meaning the actual techniques people use to discover, learn, and solve problems. She adds that "the phenomenon of risk and reassurance and our addiction to it" shows up everywhere, especially in the very human desires for hope and personal security.

She warns me, "In short, numbers are important, but framing may be as important as the numbers, and we have to be careful not to imply people are—or have been—foolish."

Excellent advice. People do things for many reasons, out of fear, out of respect for a doctor, or because they need comfort and reassurance. My naïve calculus that they "just need to know all the facts" doesn't cut it.

Wendy reminded me of a quote from Dr. Cornelia Baines who, when speaking of mammography screening said, "Even with screening, some people will die, and without screening, many will be successfully treated." Wendy reminded me that many people, whether they are conscious of it or not, think it's their fault if they get a disease or if a disease progresses because they didn't get screened. But as I hope I've shown in these pages, life and health are much more complicated than that.

Many people may take comfort in screening, in feeling they are "doing what they can" to prevent disease. Certainly the corporate advertising, the disease groups, and the many professional organizations pump that message, implicitly saying that if you wait for symptoms to manifest, you're an idiot.

Now instead of routine annual checkups (which most agree are relatively useless for healthy people), the main public health messaging seems to focus on age-related screening. Screening targeted toward an age group most likely to benefit seems more sensible than the "screen early, screen often" message we're used to hearing.

You can expect as time marches on that your doctor's electronic patient records will continue to flood him with pop-ups reminding him you're due for one type of screening or another. Maybe these reminders need to be treated like signals for you to kick-start your research, arm yourself with some questions, and take the time to think about what your motivations for screening might be and to learn what independent experts recommend.

The media, advertising, and popular culture emphasize and reinforce this notion that we all have incredible amounts of control over our health and our disease processes. And if we get a disease, it is somehow our fault—we didn't live right, we smoked or drank, ate too few greens, or lounged on our couches too much. Don't let "getting screened" automatically jump onto the list of things you feel guilty about when you leave it undone.

From her research on the "What's in a Scan?" project, Wendy told me, "It's almost like people see screening as some kind of force field that protects them from even getting disease and, remarkably, the more screening some people have, the more they suffer uncertainty and fear and desire for more."

She recalls a neighbor once telling her that if it wasn't so expensive, the answer to keeping the population healthy would be to give everyone a full-body MRI every year. That would be her solution to eliminating disease and death. If only life were that simple.

When someone is offering me something that they promise will be good for me, I like to think of the aphorism: "Don't ask a barber if you need a haircut." However much we strenuously proclaim our independence, all kinds of biases—including financial and peer group influences—can shape our interpretation of the service or product we deliver. Physicians want to do the best they can for their patients but they are also humans with a very human tendency to focus on the potential benefits and not the limitations, costs, or harms of their offerings. Learn what the independent experts say—those not motivated by the same forces as physicians or their professional bodies—and find a sound interpretation of the numbers so that you can at least understand your statistical chances of benefit and harm.

There I am, back to the numbers again.

Prior to my experience in the optometrist's chair, I wondered why people didn't ask more questions when confronted with a screening test. Now I know. It's hard to say no when you're there, already sitting in the chair. And that's why you need to do your research and be ready with your questions.

So if you're healthy, without any worrisome symptoms, and facing screening of your blood, your genes, your bones, or your mental state, remind yourself you've got one thing on your side: time. Screening is not an emergency procedure: If it is being urgently thrust upon you, you need to demand time to ask questions and probe answers.

I took my son to the orthodontist recently. His 12-year-old jaw may not have enough space to accommodate a new tooth sprouting up. No one can read the future and tell me precisely how that tooth will look in his mouth as an adult. My common sense tells me his jaw still has some growing to do, but I felt my "common sense" get beaten down, no match for an orthodontist's "professional judgment." After examining my son and giving me a long explanation of why my son needed braces sooner rather than later, the orthodontist asked my son if he had any questions.

He had one: "What happens if I do nothing?"

I was proud of him. Maybe, over the years, he was actually listening to some of my fatherly advice. That's about the most useful thing you can ask when someone is offering a medical procedure, a drug, or a screening test.

It shouldn't signal the end of the subject, but herald the beginning of a conversation.

BIBLIOGRAPHY

Agency for Health Research and Quality. "Guide to Clinical Preventive
   Services, 2010–2011." www.ahrq.gov/clinic/pocketgd1011/gcp1os2.htm.

Canadian Task Force on Preventive Health Care. www.canadiantaskforce.ca/.

Alan Cassels, Jaclyn Van Wiltenburg, and Wendy Armstrong. "What's in a
   Scan: How Well Are Consumers Informed about the Benefits and Harms
   Related to Screening Technology (CT and PET scans) in Canada?" Ottawa:
   Canadian Centre for Policy Alternatives, 2009.

Devra Davis. *The Secret History of the War on Cancer.* New York: Basic Books,
   2007.

Imogen Evans, Hazel Thornton, and Iain Chalmers. *Testing Treatments: Better
   Research for Better Healthcare.* London: The British Library, 2006 and
   2011 editions. Available at www.jameslindlibrary.org.

Nortin M. Hadler. *Rethinking Aging: Growing Old and Living Well in an Overtreated
   Society.* Chapel Hill: University of North Carolina Press, 2011.

————. *Worried Sick: A Prescription for Health in an Overtreated America.* Chapel
   Hill: University of North Carolina Press, 2008.

Adam Hedgecoe. *The Politics of Personalised Medicine: Pharmacogenetics in the Clinic.*
   Cambridge: Cambridge University Press, 2005.

Alan S. Morrison. *Screening in Chronic Disease.* Oxford University Press, 1985.

Ray Moynihan and Alan Cassels. *Selling Sickness: How the World's Biggest
   Pharmaceutical Companies Are Turning Us All into Patients.* Vancouver:
   Greystone Books, 2005.

Angela Raffle and Muir Gray. *Screening: Evidence and Practice.* New York: Oxford
   University Press, 2007.

Harriet Rosenberg and Danielle Allard. "Evidence for Caution: Women and Statin Use." Toronto: Women and Health Protection, June 2007. Available at www.whp-apsf.ca/pdf/statinsEvidenceCaution.pdf.

Gillian Sanson. *The Myth of Osteoporosis: What Every Woman Should Know about Creating Bone Health*. Ann Arbor: MCD Century Publications, 2003.

Mark Scholz and Ralph Blum. *Invasion of the Prostate Snatchers*. New York: Other Press, 2010.

United States Preventative Services Task Force. www.ahrq.gov/clinic/uspstfix.htm.

H. Gilbert Welch. *Should I Be Tested for Cancer? Maybe Not and Here's Why*. Berkeley: University of California Press, 2004.

Steven Woloshin, Lisa M. Schwartz, and H. Gilbert Welch. *Know Your Chances: Understanding Health Statistics*. Berkeley: University of California Press, 2008.

―――. *Overdiagnosed: Making People Sick in the Pursuit of Health*. Boston: Beacon Press, 2011.

J.M.G. Wilson and G. Jungner. *Principles and Practices of Screening for Disease*. Geneva: World Health Organization, 1968. Available at whqlibdoc.who.int/php/WHO_PHP_34.pdf.

ENDNOTES

PROLOGUE: *Seek and ye shall find*
1. I. Heath, "In Defence of a National Sickness Service: A Reconstituted NHS that Prioritises Prevention of Sickness Would Fail All Those Who Are Ill Now," *BMJ*, vol. 334, 2007.

CHAPTER 1: *The whole body scan: Who's really reaping the benefits, and why you don't need one*
1. Jim Wilson, "Insides Out," *Popular Mechanics*, July 2002, pp. 82–85. books. google.ca/books?id=RM8DAAAAMBAJ&pg=PA82&lpg=PA82&dq=from+the +Starship+Enterprise+to+your+local+mall&source=bl&ots=JOCKU9IYuA& sig=J2DyxhuLokGckTcbuvcqqgzJDxA&hl=en&ei=W33mTujaLrPO2WX7y4i_ BA&sa=X&oi=book_result&ct=result&resnum=1&ved=0CB4Q6AEWAA#v =onepage&q=from%20the%20Starship%20Enterprise%20to%20your%20 local%20mall&f=false (accessed January 12, 2012).
2. A. Cassels, J. van Wiltenburg, and W. Armstrong, "What's in a Scan? How Well Are Consumers Informed about the Benefits and Harms Related to Screening Technology (CT and PET scans) in Canada?" Canadian Centre for Policy Alternatives, Ottawa, April 2, 2009 (available at www.policyalternatives.ca/ publications/reports/whats-scan).
3. C.D. Furtado, D.A. Aguirre, C.B. Sirlin, et al., "Whole-Body CT Screening: Spectrum of Findings and Recommendations in 1192 Patients," *Radiology*, vol. 237, 2005, pp. 385–94. radiology.rsna.org/content/237/2/385.full (accessed January 13, 2012).
4. A. Elliott, Committee on Medical Aspects of Radiation in the Environment (COMARE), 12th report: "The Impact of Personally Initiated X-Ray Computed Tomography Scanning for the Health Assessment of Asymptomatic Individuals," Health Protection Agency for the Committee on Medical Aspects of Radiation in the Environment, 2007, p. 22.

5. D.J .Brenner and C.D. Elliston, "Estimated Radiation Risks Potentially Associated with Full Body CT Screening," *Radiology*, vol. 232, 2004, pp. 735–38. www.columbia.edu/~djb3/papers/radiol3.pdf (accessed January 13, 2012).

6. D.A. Johnson, P.R. Helft, and D.K. Rex, "CT and Radiation-Related Cancer Risk—Time for a Paradigm Shift?" (Opinion), *Nature*, vol. 6, December 2009, pp. 738–740. www.nature.com/nrgastro/journal/v6/n12/pdf/nrgastro.2009. 184.pdf (accessed January 13, 2012).

7. L. Berlin, "Potential Legal Ramifications of Whole-Body CT Screening: Taking a Peek into Pandora's Box," *American Journal of Roentgenology*, vol. 180, 2002, pp. 317–22. www.ajronline.org/cgi/reprint/180/2/317 (accessed January 13, 2012).

8. R. Al-Shahi Salman, W.N. Whiteley, C. Warlow, et al., "Screening Using Whole-Body Magnetic Resonance Imaging Scanning: Who Wants an Incidentaloma?" *Journal of Medical Screening*, vol.14, no. 1, 2007, pp. 2–4.

9. M.T. Beinfeld, E.Wittenberg, and G.S. Gazelle, "Cost Effectiveness of Whole-Body CT Screening," *Radiology*, vol. 234, 2005, pp. 415–22. radiology.rsna.org/content/234/2/415.full (accessed January 13, 2013).

10. USFDA, "Full-Body CT Scans: What You Need to Know." www.fda.gov/Radiation-EmittingProducts/RadiationEmittingProductsandProcedures/MedicalImaging/MedicalX-Rays/ucm115340.htm (accessed January 13, 2012).

11. Ibid.

12. "Doctors attack 'misleading' claims of private health screening tests," *Telegraph*, June 24, 2010. www.telegraph.co.uk/health/healthnews/7850262/Doctors-attack-misleading-claims-of-private-health-screening-tests.html (accessed January 13, 2012).

13. Author's interview with S. Woloshin and L. Schwartz, August 2008.

14. L.M. Schwartz, S. Woloshin, F.J. Fowler, Jr., et al., "Enthusiasm for Cancer Screening in the United States," *JAMA*, vol. 291, no. 1, 2004, pp. 71–78, jama. ama-assn.org/cgi/content/full/291/1/71 (accessed January 13, 2012).

15. B.M. Bauman, E.H. Chen, A.M. Mills, L. Glaspey, N.M. Thompson, M.K. Jones, and M.C. Farner, "Patient Perceptions of Computed Tomographic Imaging and Their Understanding of Radiation Risk and Exposure," *Annals of Emergency Medicine*, vol. 58, issue 1, 2010, pp. 1–7.e2. www.annemergmed.com/article/S0196-0644(10)01716-6/fulltext (accessed January 13, 2012).

16. D.J. Brenner and E.J. Hall, "Computed Tomography—An Increasing Source of Radiation Exposure," *N Engl J Med*, vol. 357, 2007, pp. 2277–84. www.nejm.org/doi/full/10.1056/NEJMra072149 (accessed January 13, 2012).

17. Electron-beam CT is used to screen for undetected coronary artery disease. Low-dose spiral CT is used to screen for cancer in the lungs and other organs. CT scans can cost between $300 and $1,000. Lee, T.H. and Brennan, T.A. "Direct-to-consumer marketing of high-technology screening tests." *New England Journal of Medicine*, vol. 346, no. 7, 2002, pp. 529–31.

18. Schwartz, et al., "Enthusiasm for cancer screening in the United States," *JAMA*, vol. 291, 2004, pp. 71–78. jama.ama-assn.org/content/291/1/71.full.pdf+htm (accessed January 13, 2012).

19. A. Cassels, et al., "What's in a Scan? How Well Are Consumers Informed about the Benefits and Harms Related to Screening Technology (CT and Pet Scans) in Canada?" Canadian Centre for Policy Alternatives, Ottawa, April 2, 2009 (available at www.policyalternatives.ca/publications/reports/ whats-scan).

20. www.oprah.com/health/How-Women-Can-Prevent-Heart-Disease-Womens-Health/1 (accessed January 12, 2012).

21. A. Elliott, "Committee on Medical Aspects of Radiation in the Environment (COMARE), 12th report: The impact of personally initiated X-ray computed tomography scanning for the health assessment of asymptomatic individuals," Health Protection Agency for the Committee on Medical Aspects of Radiation in the Environment, 2007, p. 24. Elliott notes: "There is a general consensus from the international radiology community that whole body CT scanning is not to be recommended. In particular, the following organizations have issued statements advising against the use of whole body CT scanning: American Medical Association (2005) American College of Radiology (2002) American College of Cardiology/American Heart Association (2000) American Association of Physicists in Medicine (AAPM) (2002) U.S. Agency for Healthcare Research (2005) U.S. Health Physics Society (2003) U.S. Food and Drug Administration (2002) NSW Environment Protection Authority (2003) Australia and New Zealand Health and Safety Advisory Council (2002) Radiation Advisory Council of Australia (2003) Royal Australian and New Zealand College of Radiologists (2002) College of Radiology, Academy of Medicine of Malaysia (2005)."

22. H.O. Stolberg, "Yuppie Scans from Head to Toe: Unethical Entrepreneurism," *Canadian Association of Radiologists Journal*, vol. 54, no. 1, 2003, pp. 10–3.

23. S. Gottlieb, "U.S. Commercial Scanning Clinics Are Closing Down," *BMJ*, vol. 330, 2005, p. 272. www.ncbi.nlm.nih.gov/pmc/articles/PMC548198/ (accessed January 13, 2012).

24. N. Hadler's email to author, November 27, 2011.

25. PricewaterhouseCoopers, "Medical Technology Innovation scorecard," January 2011, p. 8. www.pwc.com/us/en/health-industries/health-research-institute/innovation-scorecard (accessed January 13, 2012).

CHAPTER 2: *Screening for eyeball pressure: Know the right questions to ask (for any screening test) and when to ask them*

1. B.J. Zikmund-Fisher, M.P. Couper, E. Singer, C.A. Levin, F.J. Fowler, S. Ziniel, P.A. Ubel, and A. Fagerlin, "The DECISIONS Study: A Nationwide Survey of United States Adults Regarding 9 Common Medical Decisions, Society for Medical Decisions Making," vol. 30, no. 5, 2010, suppl 20S–34S. Originally published online April 14, 2010. The online version of this article can be found at mdm.sagepub.com/content/30/5_suppl/20S (accessed January 13, 2012).

2. The Pfizer-sponsored "All Eyes on Glaucoma" campaign urges people to get routine eye exams including tonometry: www.newswire.ca/en/story/339187/

don-t-leave-your-vision-to-chance-on-world-glaucoma-day (accessed January 16, 2012).

3. M.A. Kass, D.K Heuer, E.J. Higginbotham, C.A. Johnson, J.L. Keltner, J.P. Miller, R.K. Parrish 2nd, M.R. Wilson, and M.O.Gordon, "The Ocular Hypertension Treatment Study: A Randomized Trial Determines that Topical Ocular Hypotensive Medication Delays or Prevents the Onset of Primary Open-Angle Glaucoma." www.ncbi.nlm.nih.gov/pubmed/12049574 (accessed January 13, 2012).

4. USPSTF, "Screening for Glaucoma: Recommendation Statement." AHRQ Publication No. 04-0548-A, March 2005. www.uspreventiveservicestaskforce. org/uspstf05/glaucoma/glaucrs.pdf (accessed January 14, 2012).

5. Canadian Agency for Drugs and Technologies in Health, "Tonometry in Eye Examinations: Guidelines," January 8, 2010. www.cadth.ca/media/pdf/ K0123_Tonometry_in_eye_exams_final.pdf (accessed January 13, 2012).

6. G. Michelson and M. Groh, "Screening Models for Glaucoma," *Current Opinion in Ophthalmology*, vol. 12, no. 2, 2001, pp. 105–11.

7. M.A. Kass, D.K. Heuer, E.J. Higginbotham, et al., "The Ocular Hypertension Treatment Study: A Randomized Trial Determines that Topical Ocular Hypotensive Medication Delays or Prevents the Onset of Primary Open-Angle Glaucoma." www.ncbi.nlm.nih.gov/pubmed/12049574 (accessed January 13, 2012).

8. S. Salim, P.A. Netland, K.H. Fung, M.E. Smith, et al., "Assessment of the Student Sight Savers Program Methods for Glaucoma Screening," *Ophthalmic Epidemiology*, vol. 16, no.4, 2009, pp. 238–42. informahealthcare.com/doi/ abs/10.3109/09286580902863023 (accessed January 13, 2012).

9. D.L. Eisenberg, "Reconsidering the Gold Standard of Tonometry," *Glaucoma Today*, March 2011. bmctoday.net/glaucomatoday/2011/03/article. asp?f=reconsidering-the-gold-standard-of-tonometry (accessed January 13, 2012).

10. C.G.V. De Moraes, T.S. Prata, J. Liebmann, and R. Ritch, "Modalities of Tonometry and their Accuracy with Respect to Corneal Thickness and Irregularities," *Journal of Optometry*, vol. 1, no. 2, 2008, pp. 43–49. www.elsevier.es/sites/ default/files/elsevier/pdf/310/310v01n02a13188752pdf001.pdf (accessed January 13, 2012).

11. S. Mansberger, "Should We Be Screening for Glaucoma?" *Review of Ophthalmology*, 2010. www.revophth.com/content/d/glaucoma_management/c/22659/ (accessed January 13, 2012).

12. tonometer.wordpress.com/2010/03/04/diaton-tonometer-sponsors-world-glaucoma-day-with-free-screening-events/ (accessed January 13, 2012).

13. www.glaucoma.org/treatment/medication-guide.php (accessed January 13, 2012).

14. S.Sillino, A. Casuccio, G.M. Giammanco, C. Mammina, D. Morreale, F. Di Pace, and G. Lodato, "Tonometers and Infectious Risk: Myth or Reality? Efficacy of

Different Disinfection Regimens on Tonometer Tips," *Nature*, 2005. www.nature.com/eye/journal/v21/n4/full/6702269a.html#bib22 (accessed January 13, 2012).

CHAPTER 3: *Cholesterol screening, syndrome X, and heart scanning: The risky business of screening for risk*

1. Author's interview with George Thompson, November 4, 2011.
2. N.M. Hadler, *Rethinking Aging: Growing Old and Living Well in an Overtreated Society*, University of North Carolina Press, Chapel Hill, NC, p. 26.
3. Ibid., p. 27.
4. Therapeutics Initiative, "Do Statins Have a Role in Primary Prevention?" *Therapeutics Letter*, issue 48 (APR–JUN 2003). www.ti.ubc.ca/newsletter/do-statins-have-role-primary-prevention (accessed January 13, 2012).
5. Therapeutics Initiative, "Do Statins Have a Role in Primary Prevention? An Update." *Therapeutics Letter*, issue 77 (MAR–APR 2010). www.ti.ubc.ca/letter77 (accessed January 13, 2012).
6. Author's interview with Harriet Rosenberg, November 12, 2011.
7. www.nhlbi.nih.gov/health/health-topics/topics/bdt/ (accessed January 13, 2012).
8. GIA, press release: "Global Cholesterol and Other Cardiovascular Testing Market to Reach 2.3 Billion Units by 2015, According to a New Report by Global Industry Analysts, Inc. San Jose, CA," (Vocus/PRWEB) February 9, 2011. www.prweb.com/releases/cholesterol_testing/cardiovascular_tests/prweb8121191.htm (accessed January 13, 2012).
9. V.L. Roger, A.S. Go, D.M. Lloyd-Jones, et al., on behalf of the American Heart Association Statistics Committee and Stroke Statistics Subcommittee, "Heart Disease and Stroke Statistics—2011 Update: A Report from the American Heart Association," *Circulation*, vol. 123, no. 4, 2011, e18–e209. Epub 2010 Dec 15.
10. The International Diabetes Federation defines syndrome X as obesity joined with raised triglycerides, reduced HDL cholesterol, high blood pressure, and high blood sugars (also called increased fasting blood sugar). The World Health Organization (WHO) says if you've got "impaired glucose tolerance" (diabetes symptoms) along with two of these symptoms—high blood pressure, high cholesterol, obesity, or microalbuminemia (protein in your urine indicating kidney problems)—then you have the disease. Other definitions also abound.
11. N. Sattar, A. McConnachie, A.G. Shaper, et al., "Can Metabolic Syndrome Usefully Predict Cardiovascular Disease and Diabetes? Outcome Data from Two Prospective Studies," *The Lancet*, Volume 371, Issue 9628, 2008, pp. 1927–35. doi:10.1016/S0140-6736(08)60602-9.
12. The cutoff used to be 8 percent, then was lowered to 7 percent, and then with more intensive monitoring, to 6 percent, when the U.S. government halted a major trial of intensively lowering blood sugar levels in diabetics because too

many people were dying. See the ACCORD (Action to Control Cardiovascular Risk in Diabetes) trial press release at public.nhlbi.nih.gov/newsroom/home/GetPressRelease.aspx?id=2551 (accessed January 13, 2012).

13. N. Hadler, *Worried Sick: A Prescription for Health in an Overtreated America*, University of North Carolina Press, Chapel Hill, NC, 2008, p. 48.

14. J. Breitstein, "The Making of a New Disease," *Pharmaceutical Executive*, January 1, 2004. pharmexec.findpharma.com/pharmexec/article/articleDetail.jsp?id=80917 (accessed January 16, 2011).

15. S. Sayare, "Scandal over Mediator, a French Weight-Loss Drug, Prompts Calls for Wide Changes," *New York Times*, December 11, 2011. www.nytimes.com/2011/12/12/health/scandal-widens-over-french-weight-loss-drug-mediator.html?pagewanted=all (accessed January 13, 2012).

16. G.M. Reaven, "The Metabolic Syndrome: Is this Diagnosis Necessary?" *Am J Clin Nutr.*, vol. 83, no. 6, 2006, pp. 1237–47.

17. www.canadadiagnostic.com/screening-exams-ct-heart.php (accessed January 13, 2012).

18. Canadian Diagnostic Centre, Vancouver, brochure on website at www.canada-diagnostic.com/content/services/Atheroslcerosis_Screening.php (accessed January 13, 2012).

19. www.canadadiagnostic.com/Documents/Misc/QA-Heart-Scans.pdf (accessed January 13, 2012).

20. www.ahrq.gov/clinic/cvd/chdprovider.htm (accessed January 13, 2012).

21. J.W. McEvoy, M.J. Blaha, K. Nasir, Y.E. Yoon, E.K. Choi, I.S.Cho, E.J. Chun, S.I. Choi, J.J. Rivera, R.S. Blumenthal, and H.J. Chang. "Impact of coronary computed tomographic angiography results on patient and physician behavior in a low-risk population," *Arch Intern Med.*, vol. 171, no. 14, 2011, pp. 1260–68. Epub 2011 May 23. www.ncbi.nlm.nih.gov/pubmed/21606093 <www.ncbi.nlm.nih.gov/pubmed/21606093 (accessed January 14, 2012).

22. Author's interview with Dr. John McEvoy, June 24, 2011.

CHAPTER 4: PSA *testing: What are the odds?*

1. Author's interview with Bob Bossin, November 2011.

2. Ibid.

3. American Cancer Society, "Lifetime Risk of Developing or Dying From Cancer." www.cancer.org/Cancer/CancerBasics/lifetime-probability-of-developing-or-dying-from-cancer (accessed January 14, 2012).

4. The American Urological Association Foundation, "What You Should Know about Prostate Cancer Screening," AUA Foundation, 2009. www.auanet.org/content/media/psa1.pdf (accessed January 13, 2012).

5. American Cancer Society, "Can Prostate Cancer Be Found Early?" www.cancer.org/Cancer/ProstateCancer/DetailedGuide/prostate-cancer-detection (accessed January 13, 2012).

6. R. Chou, J.M. Croswell, T. Dana, et al., "Screening for Prostate Cancer: A Review of the Evidence for the U.S. Preventive Services Task Force," U.S. Preventive

Services Task Force, October 7, 2011. www.uspreventiveservicestaskforce.org/
uspstf12/prostate/prostateart.htm (accessed January 13, 2012).

7. R.K. Nam, R. Saskin, Y. Lee, et al., "Increasing Hospital Admission Rates
for Urological Complications after Transrectal Ultrasound Guided Prostate
Biopsy," *J Urol.*, vol. 183, no. 3, 2010, pp. 963–68, Epub 2010 Jan 20.
www.ncbi.nlm.nih.gov/pubmed/20089283 (accessed January 13, 2012).

8. S. Loeb, H. Ballentine Carter, S.I. Berndt, et al., "Complications after Prostate
Biopsy: Data from SEER-Medicare," *The Journal of Urology*, vol. 186, issue 5, 2011,
pp. 1830–34,. DOI: 10.1016/j.juro.2011.06.057). www.jurology.com/article/
S0022-5347(11)04336-9/abstract (accessed January 12, 2012).

9. F.H. Schröder, J. Hugosson, M.J. Roobol, et al., for the ERSPC Investigators,
"Screening and Prostate-Cancer Mortality in a Randomized European Study,"
N Engl J Med, vol. 360, 2009, pp. 1320–28. www.nejm.org/doi/full/10.1056/
NEJMoa0810084 (accessed January 13, 2012).

10. J. Hegarty, P.V. Beirne, E. Walsh, H. Comber, T. Fitzgerald, and M. Wallace
Kazer, "Radical Prostatectomy versus Watchful Waiting for Prostate Cancer,"
Cochrane Summaries, November 10, 2010. summaries.cochrane.org/
CD006590/radical-prostatectomy-rp-versus-watchful-waiting-ww-for-the-
treatment-of-localized-prostate-cancer-a-review-of-the-evidence (accessed
January 13, 2012).

11. L. Holmberg, A. Bill-Axelson, F. Helgesen, J.O. Salo, P. Folmerz, M. Häggman,
et al., "A Randomised Trial Comparing Radical Prostatectomy with Watchful
Waiting in Early Prostate Cancer," *The New England Journal of Medicine*, vol. 347,
no. 11, 2002, pp. 781–89. E. Johansson, A. Bill-Axelson, L. Holmberg, E. Onelöv,
J.-E. Johanssson, and G. Steineck, for the Scandinavian Prostate Cancer Group,
"Time, Symptom Burden, Androgen Deprivation and Self-Assessed Quality
of Life after Radical Prostatectomy or Watchful Waiting: The Randomized
Scandinavian Prostate Cancer Group Study Number 4 (SPCG-4) Clinical Trial,"
European Urology, vol. 55, 2009, pp. 422–32.

12. J. Hegarty, P.V. Beirne, E. Walsh, H. Comber, T. Fitzgerald, and M. Wallace
Kazer, "Radical Prostatectomy versus Watchful Waiting for Prostate Cancer
(Review)," *The Cochrane Library*, Issue 11, 2010. www.update-software.com/BCP/
WileyPDF/EN/CD006590.pdf. The exact phrasing was "This single trial does
not provide sufficient evidence to allow confident statements to be made about
the magnitude of any beneficial and harmful effects of RP compared with WW
for men with clinically detected prostate cancers."

13. J.L. Stanford, Z. Feng, A.S. Hamilton, F.D. Gilliland, R.A. Stephenson, J.W. Eley,
et al., "Urinary and Sexual Function after Radical Prostatectomy for Clinically
Localized Prostate Cancer: The Prostate Cancer Outcomes Study," *JAMA*,
vol. 283, 2000, pp. 354–60.

14. Author's interview with Calvin Cairns, December 2011.

15. A. Raffle and M. Gray, *Screening: Evidence and Practice*, Oxford University Press,
2007, p. 68.

16. Zero: The project to end prostate cancer, press release, "Zero Works With Congress to Protect Early Detection," November 21, 2011. zerocancer.org/news/releases/zero-works-with-congress-to-protect-early-detection/ (accessed January 14, 2012).

17. Depends website at www.depend.com, "Ten Questions to Ask Your Doctor about Prostate Cancer." www.depend.com/caring-for-others/articles/10-questions-to-ask-the-doctor-about-prostate-cancer/14000000505 (accessed January 13, 2012).

18. Ibid.

19. www.clarosdx.com/documents/Start-Up-Claros-07.pdf (accessed January 13, 2012).

20. E. Licking and R. Longman, "Molecular Diagnostics—From Tools to Tests," *IN VIVO*, vol. 24, no. 5, May 2006.

21. One company, Mediwatch Plc, is a urological diagnostic company, which has a worldwide distribution of PSAwatch, its flagship point-of-care total PSA measuring system for prostate cancer. Mediawatch, "Five Year Global Distribution Agreement Secured." www.mediwatch.com/NewsDetail.php?articleId=134 (accessed January 13, 2012).

22. Author's interview with Dr. Mark Scholz, November 2011.

23. D.V. Makarov, J.B. Yu, R.A. Desai, D.F. Penson, and C.P. Gross, "The Association between Diffusion of the Surgical Robot and Radical Prostatectomy Rates," *Medical Care*, vol. 49, no. 4, 2011, pp. 333–39. journals.lww.com/lww-medicalcare/Abstract/2011/04000/The_Association_Between_Diffusion_of_the_Surgical.1.aspx (accessed January 13, 2012).

24. H.G. Welch, S. Woloshin, and L. Schwartz, *Overdiagnosed: Making People Sick in the Pursuit of Health*, Beacon Press, Boston, 2011, p. 60.

25. "Prostate Cancer Drug Market Forecast to Grow from $3.6 Billion in 2010 to $10.1 Billion in 2020," November 7, 2011. www.news-medical.net/news/20111107/Prostate-cancer-drug-market-forecast-to-grow-from-2436-billion-in-2010-to-24101-billion-in-2020.aspx (accessed January 13, 2012).

26. R.J. Ablin, "The Great Prostate Mistake," *New York Times*, March 9, 2010, p. A27.

27. J.D. Voss and J.M. Schectman, "Prostate Cancer Screening Practices and Beliefs: A Longitudinal Physician Survey," *Journal of General Internal Medicine*, vol. 16, no. 12, 2001, pp. 831–37. doi: 10.1111/j.1525-1497.2001.10133.x. www.ncbi.nlm.nih.gov/pmc/articles/PMC1495300/ (accessed January 14, 2012).

28. A. Peticolas, "Conductors on a One-Way Track: Do Medical Authorities Really Get to Decide Policy About Medical Screening Tests?" Medscape General Medicine™, posted May 5, 2003. www.medscape.com/viewarticle/452598.

29. M.H. Farrell, M.A. Murphy, and C.E. Schneider, "How Underlying Patient Beliefs Can Affect Physician-Patient Communication about Prostate-Specific Antigen Testing." *Eff Clin Pract*, vol. 5, no. 3, 2002, pp. 120–29.

30. National Cancer Institute, "Factsheet on Prostate Cancer." www.cancer.gov/cancertopics/factsheet/detection/PSA#a3 (accessed January 13, 2012).

CHAPTER 5: *Mammography screening: The politics, the promises, and the numbers*

1. Author's interview with Mary Brown, July 2011.
2. Canadian Task Force on Preventive Health Care, "Screening for Breast Cancer: Summary of Recommendations for Clinicians and Policy-Makers." www.canadiantaskforce.ca/recommendations/2011_01_eng.html (accessed January 14, 2012).
3. K. Doheny, "Canadian Guidelines Support No Routine Mammograms until 50," USA *Today*, November 21, 2011. yourlife.usatoday.com/health/medical/breastcancer/story/2011-11-22/Canadian-guidelines-support-no-routine-mammograms-until-50/51346478/1 (accessed January 14, 2012).
4. American College of Radiology, "New National Poll: 89 Percent of Women Said Mammograms Vital to Their Health," September 27, 2011. www.acr.org/MainMenuCategories/media_room/FeaturedCategories/BreastImaging/89-Percent-of-Women-Said-Mammograms-Vital-to-Their-Health.aspx (accessed January 14, 2012).
5. D. Mavroforou, et al., "Screening Mammography, Public Perceptions, and Medical Liability," *European Journal of Radiology*, vol. 57, issue 3, pp. 428–35. A.
6. C.J. Baines, "Rethinking Breast Screening—Again," BMJ, vol. 331(7523), 2005, p. 1031. PMCID: PMC1273473.
7. National Cancer Institute website, "Screening Mammography: Help with Explaining Benefits and Potential Harms." www.cancer.gov/cancertopics/screening/breast/mammography-benefits-harms (accessed January 14, 2012).
8. Canadian Breast Cancer Foundation website, "Detecting Breast Cancer Earlier." www.cbcf.org/bc/AboutBreastHealth/EarlyDetection/Pages/default.aspx (accessed January 14, 2012).
9. Canadian Breast Cancer Foundation website, "Breast Screening Technology." www.cbcf.org/bc/AboutBreastHealth/EarlyDetection/Pages/Breast-Screening-Technology.aspx (accessed January 14, 2012).
10. L. Schwartz, S. Woloshin, and H.G. Welch, *Know Your Chances: Understanding Health Statistics*, University of California Press, Berkeley, CA, 2008.
11. The Canadian Task Force on Preventive Health Care, "Recommendations on Screening for Breast Cancer in Average-Risk Women Aged 40–74 years," CMAJ, vol. 183, no. 17, 2011. doi: 10.1503/cmaj.110334.
12. H.G. Welch, W.C. Black, "Overdiagnosis in Cancer," J Natl Cancer Inst, vol. 102, 2010, pp. 605–13. jnci.oxfordjournals.org/content/102/9/605.full (accessed January 14, 2012).
13. Ibid.
14. K.J. Jørgensen and P.C. Gøtzsche, "Overdiagnosis in Publicly Organised Mammography Screening Programmes: Systematic Review of Incidence Trends," BMJ, vol. 339, 2009, b2587.
15. The Canadian Task Force on Preventive Health Care, "Recommendations on Screening for Breast Cancer in Average-Risk Women Aged 40–74 Years," CMAJ, vol. 183, no. 17, 2011. doi: 10.1503/cmaj.110334.

16. Canadian Cancer Society, "Canadian Statistics on Cancer, 2008." www.quebec. cancer.ca/quebec/communiques/Stats08_FicheFaitsBref_en.pdf (accessed January 14, 2012).

17. P. Autier, M. Boniol, A. Gavin, and L.J. Vatten, "Breast Cancer Mortality in Neighbouring European Countries with Different Levels of Screening but Similar Access to Treatment: Trend Analysis of WHO Mortality Database," *BMJ*, vol. 343, 2011, d4411. www.bmj.com/content/343/bmj.d4411 (accessed January 14, 2012).

18. C.J. Baines, "Frank Words about Breast Screening," *Open Medicine*, vol. 5, no. 3, 2011, e134-36. www.openmedicine.ca/article/viewArticle/461/416 (accessed January 14, 2012).

19. D. Davis, *The Secret History on the War on Cancer*, Basic Books, New York, 2007, p. 79.

20. C.J. Baines,"Frank Words about Breast Screening," *Open Medicine*, vol. 5, no. 3, 2011, e134-6. www.openmedicine.ca/article/viewArticle/461/416 (accessed January 14, 2012).

CHAPTER 6: *Colon and cervix screening: Too much of a good thing?*

1. Biography of William Casarella, Emory University website. www.med.emory. edu/dean/casarella.cfm (accessed January 15, 2012).

2. W. J. Casarella, Letter to the editor, "A Patient's Viewpoint on a Current Controversy," *Radiology*, vol. 224, 2002, pp. 927.

3. USPSTF, www.uspreventiveservicestaskforce.org/uspstf08/colocancer/colors. htm (accessed January 15, 2012).

4. Author's interview with Dr. Casarella, November 12, 2008. Part of this interview was in the CBC radio documentary entitled *You Are Prediseased.*

5. H.G. Welch, *Overdiagnosed: Making People Sick in the Pursuit of Health*, Beacon Press, Boston, p. 95.

6. Ibid., p. 100.

7. U.S. Centers for Disease Control and Prevention, "Colon Cancer Screening Rates." www.cdc.gov/cancer/colorectal/statistics/screening_rates.htm (accessed January 15, 2012). Findings from the National Health Interview Survey (NHIS), which is administered by CDC, indicate that in 2005, only 50 percent of U.S. adults age 50 or older had undergone a sigmoidoscopy or colonoscopy within the previous 10 years or had used a fecal occult blood test (FOBT) home test kit within the preceding year.

8. H.G. Welch, *Should I Be Tested for Cancer? Maybe Not and Here's Why.* University of California Press, Berkeley, 2004, p. 40

9. H.G. Welch, *Overdiagnosed*, p. 71.

10. USPSTF, "Screening for Colorectal Cancer," October 2008. www.uspreventive-servicestaskforce.org/uspstf/uspscolo.htm (accessed January 16, 2012).

11. J.S Mandel, J.H.Bond, T.R. Church, D.C. Snover, G.M. Bradley, L.M. Schuman, and F. Ederer, "Reducing Mortality from Colorectal Cancer by Screening for

Fecal Occult Blood. Minnesota Colon Cancer Control Study." *N Engl J Med.*, vol., 328, no. 19, 1993 pp. 1365–71. www.ncbi.nlm.nih.gov/pubmed/8474513?dopt= AbstractPlus (accessed January 15, 2012).

12. American College of Radiology, press release, "ACRIN Trial Demonstrates Comparable Accuracy for CT Colonography and Standard Colonoscopy," no date. www.acr.org/MainMenuCategories/media_room/FeaturedCategories/Videos/CTC-Trial.aspx (accessed January 15, 2012).

13. B. Hendrick, "Virtual Colonoscopy a Less Invasive Cancer Screener. Scanner Images Replace Colonoscope, Lessen Patient Risk," *Atlanta Journal-Constitution*, October 8, 2008. www.ajc.com/health/content/health/stories/2008/10/08/colon_cancer_virtual_screening.html (accessed January 15, 2012).

14. Healthnewsreviews.org review of "Virtual Colonoscopy a Less Invasive Cancer Screener," October 8, 2008, a story from the *Atlanta Journal-Constitution*. Review is here: www.healthnewsreview.org/review/1552/ (accessed January 15, 2012).

15. USPSTF, "Screening for Colorectal Cancer," October 2008. www.uspreventiveservicestaskforce.org/uspstf/uspscolo.htm (accessed January 15, 2012).

16. American Cancer Society, "2011 Cancer Facts and Figures," p. 10. www.cancer.org/acs/groups/content/@epidemiologysurveilance/documents/document/acspc-029771.pdf (accessed January 15, 2012).

17. C. Dolinsky and C. Hill-Kayser. "Cervical Cancer: The Basics," Oncolink.org (Abramson Cancer Center of the University of Pennsylvania), January 16, 2011. www.oncolink.org/types/article.cfm?c=6&s=17&ss=129&id=8226&CFID=397 37627&CFTOKEN=60205964 (accessed January 15, 2012)

18. Ibid.

19. International Agency for Research on Cancer (IARC) Working Group on the Evaluation of Cervical Cancer Screening Programmes. "Screening for Squamous Cervical Cancer: Duration of Low Risk after Negative Results of Cervical Cytology and Its Implication for Screening Policies," *Br Med J*, vol. 293, no. 6548, 1986, pp. 659–64.

20. R. Sharpe and E. Lucas, "Forty Percent of Medicare Spending on Common Cancer Screenings Unnecessary, Probe Suggests," iWatch News, October 7, 2011. www.iwatchnews.org/2011/10/07/6898/forty-percent-medicare-spending-common-cancer-screenings-unnecessary-probe-suggests (accessed January 15, 2012).

21. C. S. Sima, K.S. Panageas, and D. Schrag, "Cancer Screening among Patients with Advanced Cancer," *JAMA*, vol. 304, no. 14, 2010, pp. 1584–91. doi: 10.1001/jama.2010.1449.

22. The Iwatch report is brilliant. Check it out here: www.iwatchnews.org/2011/10/07/6898/forty-percent-medicare-spending-common-cancer-screenings-unnecessary-probe-suggests (accessed January 15, 2012).

23. Julian Tudor Hart, "The Inverse Care Law," *Lancet*, vol. 297, issue 7696, 1971, pp. 405–12.

CHAPTER 7: *Mental health screening: We're crazy, just not that crazy*

1. Author's interview with Brett Thombs, October 11, 2011.
2. Columbia University TeenScreen Program, "The Columbia University TeenScreen Program: Getting Started Guide," p. 3. www.psychsearch.net/revised_getting_started_guide_final.pdf (accessed January 15, 2012).
3. Centers for Disease Control and Prevention, National Center for Injury Prevention and Control. Web-based Injury Statistics Query and Reporting System (WISQARS): www.cdc.gov/ncipc/wisqars.
4. TeenScreen National Center for Mental Health Checkups at Columbia University, "New Freedom Commission on Mental Health." www.teenscreen.org/about/support-endorsements/new-freedom-commission-on-mental-health/ (accessed January 15, 2012).
5. M. Hogan, chairman, the President's New Freedom Commission on Mental Health Report, July 22, 2003. Page 63 describes TeenScreen as a "Model Program: Screening Program for Youth" and page 69 describes TMAP as a "Model Program: Quality Medications Care for Serious Mental Illness." www.nami.org/Template.cfm?Section=New_Freedom_Commission&Template=/ContentManagement/ContentDisplay.cfm&ContentID=28335 (accessed January 15, 2012).
6. L.Ross, "Zyprexa and TeenScreen Marketing Ploys," as part of the Mindfreedom USA Campaign wrote, "The New Freedom Commission, TMAP, and TeenScreen appear to be a blatant political/pharmaceutical company alliance that promotes medication, and more precisely, the newer, more expensive antidepressants and antipsychotics which are at best, of questionable benefit and come with deadly side effects." www.mindfreedom.org/campaign/usa/zyprexa-teenscreen (accessed January 15, 2012).
7. M. Petersen, "Making Drugs, Shaping the Rules," *New York Times,* February 1, 2004. www.nytimes.com/2004/02/01/business/making-drugs-shaping-the-rules.html?scp=3&sq=&pagewanted=1 (accessed January 15, 2012).
8. "PHQ-9 Questionnaire Modified for Teens." www.teenscreen.org/wp-content/uploads/PHQ-9-Modified-read-only.pd (accessed January 15, 2012).
9. The Associated Press, "Depression Tests Urged for Teenagers," *New York Times,* March 29, 2009. www.nytimes.com/2009/03/30/health/30depression.html?scp=4&sq=mental%20health%20screening&st=cse (accessed January 15, 2012).
10. M.J.L. Kirby and W.J. Keon, "Out of the Shadows at Last: Transforming Mental Health, Mental Illness and Addiction Services in Canada," The Standing Senate Committee on Social Affairs, Science and Technology, May 2006. www.parl.gc.ca/Content/SEN/Committee/391/soci/rep/repo2mayo6part2-e.htm#_Toc133223090 (accessed January 15, 2012).
11. N. Hoffman's presentation, June 21, 2005, "Proceedings of the Standing Senate Committee." www.parl.gc.ca/Content/SEN/Committee/381/soci/23eva-e.htm?Language=E&Parl=38&Ses=1&comm_id=47 (accessed January 15, 2012).

12. M.J.L. Kirby and W.J. Keon, "Out of the Shadows at Last: Transforming Mental Health, Mental Illness and Addiction Services in Canada," the Standing Senate Committee on Social Affairs, Science and Technology, May 2006.

13. Senate Standing Committee, "Mental Health, Mental Illness and Addiction: Overview of Policies and Programs in Canada, Report 1," para. 8.2.7. www.parl. gc.ca/Content/SEN/Committee/381/soci/rep/report1/repintnovo4vol1part3-e. htm (accessed January 15, 2012).

14. Author's interview with Jo Anne Cook, November 23, 2011.

15. S. Gilbody, A. House, and T. Sheldon, "Screening and Case Finding Instruments for Depression," Cochrane Database of Systematic Reviews, 2005, Issue 4, Art. No.: CD002792. Published online: January 21, 2009. summaries.cochrane. org/CD002792/screening-and-case-finding-instruments-for-depression (accessed January 15, 2012).

16. USPSTF, "Screening for Depression," May 2002. www.uspreventiveservices-taskforce.org/uspstf/uspsdepr.htm (accessed January 15, 2012).

17. Mental Health America, "Depression Screener" at: www.depression-screening. org/depression_screen.cfm (accessed January 15, 2012).

18. IMS Health, "Top-line Market Data 2008" (U.S. Sales and Prescription Information.) www.imshealth.com/portal/site/imshealth/menuitem.a46c6d4df3db4b 3d88f611019418c22a/?vgnextoid=85f4a56216a10210vgnVCM10000oedi52c a2RCRD&cpsextcurrchannel=1 (accessed January 15, 2012).

19. Author's interview with Dr. Joel Paris, November 9, 2010.

20. M. Zimmerman, J.N. Galione, C.J. Ruggero, I. Chelminski, J.B. McGlinchey, K. Dalrymple, and D. Young, "Performance of the Mood Disorders Questionnaire in a Psychiatric Outpatient Setting," *Bipolar Disorder*, vol. 11, no. 7, 2009, pp. 759–65.

21. You only have to look at the financial disclosures in this article: G. Parker, et al., "Issues for DSM-5: Whither Melancholia? The Case for Its Classification as a Distinct Mood Disorder," *Am J Psychiatry*, vol. 167, 2010, pp. 745–47. 10.1176/ appi.ajp.2010.09101525.

CHAPTER 8: *Self-screening for disease: Planting the seeds of self-doubt*

1. D. Spence, "Bad Medicine: Adult Attention-Deficit/Hyperactivity Disorder," *BMJ*, vol. 343, 2011, d7244. doi: 10.1136/bmj.d7244 (published November 7, 2011).

2. psychcentral.com/quizzes/adultaddquiz.htm (accessed January 15, 2012).

3. Author's interview with Barbara Mintzes, November 27, 2011.

4. Author's interview with Dr. David Healy, March 1, 2011, Victoria, BC.

5. D. Healy, *Mania: A Short History of Bipolar Disorder*, Johns Hopkins University Press, Baltimore, 2011, p. 133.

6. Author's interview with Dr. David Healy, March 1, 2011, Victoria, BC.

7. D.J. Handelsman, "Testosterone and Male Ageing: Spinning the Wheels," *MJA*, vol. 193, no. 7, 2010, pp. 379–80.

8. A. Weintraub, "Testosterone is Sure Looking Virile: Despite Legal Setbacks and FDA Delays, Youth-Crazed Boomers Are Making It a Billion-Dollar Industry," Bloomberg Businessweek, September 29, 2009. www.businessweek.com/magazine/content/09_45/b4154058755602.htm (accessed January 15, 2012).

9. Abbott Pharmaceuticals, press release, "Abbott Completes Acquisition of Solvay Pharmaceuticals," February 16, 2010. www.abbott.com/news-media/press-releases/Press_Release_0819.htm (accessed January 15, 2012).

10. A. Weintraub, "Testosterone Is Sure Looking Virile: Despite Legal Setbacks and FDA Delays, Youth-Crazed Boomers Are Making It a Billion-Dollar Industry," Bloomberg Businessweek, October 29, 2009. www.businessweek.com/magazine/content/09_45/b4154058755602.htm (accessed January 15, 2012).

11. USFDA, press release, "Testosterone Gel Safety Concerns Prompt FDA to Require Label Changes, Medication Guide," May 7, 2009. www.fda.gov/News-Events/Newsroom/PressAnnouncements/2009/ucm149580.htm (accessed January 15, 2012).

12. Press release, "National Survey Shows Men Reluctant to Talk to Physicians About Low Libido, Self-Screening Tool Helps Aid Communication," June 12, 2001. thyroid.about.com/library/news/bllibido.htm (accessed January 15, 2012).

CHAPTER 9: *Lung screening for cancer and* COPD:
Finding disease in every breath you take

1. NCI, press release, "Lung Cancer Trial Results Show Mortality Benefit with Low-Dose CT: Twenty Percent Fewer Lung Cancer Deaths Seen among Those Who Were Screened with Low-Dose Spiral CT Than with Chest X-ray," November 4, 2010. www.cancer.gov/newscenter/pressreleases/2010/NLST-resultsRelease (accessed January 15, 2012).

2. For the full results: National Lung Screening Trial Research Team, "Reduced Lung-Cancer Mortality with Low-Dose Computed Tomographic Screening," *New England Journal of Medicine*, vol. 365, 2011, pp. 395–409. www.nejm.org/doi/full/10.1056/NEJMoa1102873#t=articleResults (accessed January 15, 2012).

3. USPSTF, "Lung Cancer Screening," May 2004. www.uspreventiveservicestask-force.org/uspstf/uspslung.htm (accessed January 15, 2012).

4. Centers for Disease Control, "Lung Cancer Statistics." www.cdc.gov/cancer/lung/statistics/ (accessed January 15, 2012).

5. http://www.mayfairdiagnostics.com/?setregion=Calgary (accessed February 12, 2012).

6. CBC website, "Executive Physicals 'Bad Medicine,' Journal Article Claims," October 1, 2008. www.cbc.ca/news/health/story/2008/10/01/exec-physicals-commentary.html (accessed January 15, 2012).

7. Ibid.

8. Ibid.

9. B. Rank, "Executive Physicals—Bad Medicine on Three Counts," *N Engl J Med*, vol. 359, 2008, pp. 1424–25.

10. Author's interview with Barnett Kramer, June 18, 2008.
11. Ibid., USPSTF, "Lung Cancer Screening."
12. D. Spence, "When Marketing Masquerades as Education," BMJ, vol. 342, 2011, c7469. doi: 10.1136/bmj.c7469 (published January 4, 2011).
13. USPSTF, "Screening for Chronic Obstructive Pulmonary Disease Using Spirometry Recommendation Statement," March 2008. www.uspreventiveservicestaskforce.org/uspstf08/copd/copdrs.htm (accessed January 15, 2012).
14. D. Spence, "When Marketing Masquerades as Education," BMJ, vol. 342, 2011, c7469 (published January 4, 2011) www.bmj.com/content/342/bmj.c7469 (subscription required).
15. www.knowcopd.com/copd-diagnosis.jsp (accessed January 15, 2012).

CHAPTER 10: *Bone screening: Selling screening*
1. R.S. Weinstein, P. K. Roberson, and S.C. Manolagas, "Giant Osteoclast Formation and Long-Term Oral Bisphosphonate Therapy," N Engl J Med, vol. 360, 2009, pp. 53–62. www.nejm.org/doi/full/10.1056/NEJMoa0802633#t=articleResults (accessed January 15, 2011).
2. S. Boyles, "Osteoporosis Drugs Work, but How?" WebMD Health News, December 31, 2008. www.webmd.com/osteoporosis/news/20081231/osteoporosis-drugs-work-but-how (accessed January 15, 2011).
3. D.K. Wysowski (Food and Drug Administration), "Reports of Esophageal Cancer with Oral Bisphosphonate Use," N Engl J Med, vol. 360, 2009 pp. 89–90. www.nejm.org/doi/full/10.1056/NEJMc0808738 (accessed January 15 2011).
4. P.P. Sedghizadeh, K. Stanley, M. Caligiuri, et al., "Oral Bisphosphonate Use and the Prevalence of Osteonecrosis of the Jaw: An Institutional Inquiry," J Am Dent Assoc., vol. 140, 2009, pp.61–66. www.endoexperience.com/userfiles/file/unnamed/Oral%20bisphosphonate%20use%20and%20the%20prevalence%20of%20osteonecrosis_of%20the%20jaw%202008.pdf (accessed January 15, 2011).
5. C.J. Green, K. Bassett, V. Foerster, and A. Kazanjian, "Bone Mineral Density Testing: Does the Evidence Support Its Selective Use in Well Women?" Vancouver: University of British Columbia, 1997. British Columbia Office of Health Technology Assessment report no. 97:2T.
6. "Osteoporosis Drug Market to Grow to US$14 Billion By 2014," December 5, 2006. www.redorbit.com/news/health/755741/osteoporosis_drug_market_to_grow_to_us14_billion_by_2014/index.html (accessed January 15, 2011).
7. Author's interview with Dr. Ken Bassett, various dates. Information confirmed with Dr. Bassett on January 6, 2012.
8. D.M. Black, S.R. Cummings, D.B. Karpf, et al., "Randomised Trial of Effect of Alendronate on Risk of Fracture In Women with Existing Vertebral Fractures," Lancet, vol. 348, 1996, pp. 1535–41. www.thelancet.com/journals/lancet/article/PIIS0140-6736(96)07088-2/fulltext (accessed January 15, 2011).

9. G. Sanson, "Esophageal Cancer, Jaw Bone Necrosis, and Giant Floating Osteo-clasts!" Weblog: Evidence-Based Perspectives on Hot Women's Health Issues, January 5, 2009. gilliansanson.wordpress.com/ (accessed January 15, 2011).
10. B. Abrahamsen, P. Eiken, and R. Eastell, "Sub-trochanteric and Diaphyseal Femur Fractures in Patients Treated with Alendronate: A Register-Based National Cohort Study," JBMR, vol. 24, no. 6, 2009, pp. 1095–102. doi: 10.1359/JBMR.081247.
11. G. Sanson, "Esophageal Cancer, Jaw Bone Necrosis, and Giant Floating Osteo-clasts!" Weblog: Evidence-Based Perspectives on Hot Women's Health Issues, January 5, 2009. gilliansanson.wordpress.com/ (accessed January 15, 2011).
12. G. Sanson, "New Osteoporosis Diagnostic Guidelines: A Minefield to Negoti-ate," Weblog: Evidence-Based Perspectives on Hot Women's Health Issues, June 1, 2011. gilliansanson.wordpress.com/ (accessed January 15, 2011).

CHAPTER 11: *Gene screening: When marketing precedes science*

1. 23andMe, press release, "23andMe Database Surpasses 100,000 Users," June 15, 2011. www.23andme.com/about/press/23andme_database_100000k_users/ (accessed January 15, 2012).
2. Now available on YouTube at www.youtube.com/watch?v=JT1Y310FGBU (accessed January 15, 2012).
3. European Society of Human Genetics, "Statement of the ESHG on Direct-to-Consumer Genetic Testing for Health-Related Purposes," *European Journal of Human Genetics*, August 25, 2010. doi:10.1038/ejhg.2010.129. www.eshg.org/fileadmin/www.eshg.org/documents/PPPC/2010-ejhg2010129a.pdf (accessed January 15, 2012).
4. Submission by GeneWatch U.K. to the U.K. House of Commons Health Committee, "Influence of the Pharmaceutical Industry," 4th Report of session 2004–2005, Volume II, p. 74. www.publications.parliament.uk/pa/cm200405/cmselect/cmhealth/42/42.pdf (accessed January 15, 2012).
5. Well documented in Helen Wallace, "Big Tobacco and the Human Genome: Driving the Scientific Bandwagon?" *Genomics, Society and Policy* 2009, vol. 5, no. 1, pp. 1–54. www.hss.ed.ac.uk/genomics/documents/Vol5No1.pdf (accessed January 15, 2012).
6. *Time* magazine (January 15, 2001) cover had a picture of a double-helix DNA molecule inside a prescription bottle, with the words, "Drugs of the Future: Amazing New Medicines Will Be Based on DNA. Find Out How They Will Change Your Life." www.time.com/time/covers/0,16641,20010115,00.html (accessed January 15, 2012). The January 18, 2010, cover read, "Why Your DNA Is Not Your Destiny." www.time.com/time/covers/0,16641,20100118,00.html (accessed January 15, 2012).
7. GeneWatch, press release, "GeneWatch U.K. Welcomes Rejection of 'Bar-Coding Babies' Plan," March 31, 2005. www.genewatch.org/article.shtml?als%5BCid%5D=568490&als%5Bitemid%5D=507897 (accessed January 15, 2012).

8. Huntington's Disease Society of America, "What is Huntington's Disease (H.D.)?" www.hdsa.org/about/our-mission/what-is-hd.html (accessed January 15, 2012).

9. Author's interview with Bev Heim-Myers, June 28, 2011.

10. www.ncbi.nlm.nih.gov/pmc/articles/PMC2694258/ (accessed January 15, 2012).

11. M. Evans, "DNA Database Created from Babies' Blood Samples," *Telegraph*, May 23, 2010. www.telegraph.co.uk/health/7756320/DNA-database-created-from-babies-blood-samples.html (accessed November 11, 2011).

12. Author's interview with Jason Gratl, February 2011.

13. GeneWatch press release, "Nobel Prizewinners, Tobacco Funding and the Human Genome," no date. www.genewatch.org/article.shtml?als%5Bcid%5D=492860&als%5Bitemid%5D=566452 (accessed January 15, 2012).

14. A. Picard, " 'Alarming' Rise in Dementia Comes with a Crippling Price Tag," *Globe and Mail*, September 21, 2010. www.theglobeandmail.com/life/health/dementia/alarming-rise-in-dementia-comes-with-a-crippling-price-tag/article1715781/ (accessed January 15, 2012).

15. Alzheimer's Disease International: www.alz.co.uk/ (accessed January 15, 2012).

16. Alzheimer's Disease International, "World Alzheimer's Report 2011," www.alz.co.uk/research/world-report-2011 (accessed January 15, 2012).

17. Alzheimer's Disease International, "World Alzheimer's Report 2011: The Benefits of Early Diagnosis and Intervention," Executive Summary, p. 3. www.alz.co.uk/research/WorldAlzheimerReport2011ExecutiveSummary.pdf (accessed January 15, 2012).

18. Ibid., p. 16.

19. Ibid.

20. J.W. Williams, B.L. Plassman, J.Burke, T. Holsinger, and S. Benjamin, "Preventing Alzheimer's Disease and Cognitive Decline. Evidence," Report/Technology Assessment Number 193, Agency for Healthcare Research and Quality, U.S. Department of Health and Human Services. www.ahrq.gov/downloads/pub/evidence/pdf/alzheimers/alzcog.pdf (accessed January 15, 2012).

21. Alzheimer's Society of Canada brochure, "Alzheimer's Disease and Related Dementias: The Importance of Early Diagnosis." www.alzheimer.ca/en/About-dementia/For-health-care-professionals/~/media/Files/national/pdfs/English/Brochures/EarlydiagnosisEnglishFINAL.ashx (accessed January 15, 2012).

22. D. Wilson, "Lilly Stops Alzheimer's Drug Trials," *New York Times*, August 17, 2010. www.nytimes.com/2010/08/18/business/18lilly.html (accessed January 15, 2012).

ACKNOWLEDGMENTS

I DEDICATE this book to my father, Earle Cassels, who died in 1986, four months too early to see me graduate from the Royal Military College of Canada. Back in the 1980s, doctors, looking for lung cancer, ordered routine chest X-rays as part of the annual physical, especially if you were a smoker. Even though we'll never know if it was the cancer or the complications from the surgery to remove a "spot'" on his lung that lead to my father's death, the fact that doctors no longer order routine chest X-rays on healthy patients gives me a ray of hope that the world is evolving, that screening recommendations over time are becoming more rational, cautious, and thoughtful. I hope my book accelerates that evolution.

The world's understanding of screening and overdiagnosis took a huge leap forward recently with the work of Drs. H. Gilbert Welch, Lisa Schwartz, and Steve Woloshin, and I owe many thanks to their inspiration and careful scholarship. Other heavyweights whose writings and thoughts have influenced me greatly include Cornelia Baines, William Casarella, Muir Gray, Nortin Hadler, David Healy, Bev Heim-Myers, Don Husereau, Barnett Kramer, Barbara Mintzes, Joel Paris, Harriet Rosenberg, Mark Scholz, Des Spence, Brett Thombs, Marcello Tonelli, Helen Wallace, and many members, too numerous to mention, of the internationally acclaimed Cochrane Collaboration.

Among my friends, interviewees, and colleagues, who have been incredibly generous with their time, support, and inspiration I have to thank Wendy Armstrong, Lynne Bain, Ken Bassett, Dave Beers, Warren Bell, Bob Bossin, Calvin Cairns, Maliya Cassels, Jo Ann Cook, Colin Dormuth, Kathleen Flaherty, Juan Gervas, David Henry, Andrew Macleod, Malcolm Maclure, Frederick Mikelberg, Jaclyn Morrison, Ray Moynihan, Maryann Napoli, Kerry Patriarche, Harriet Rosenberg, Gary Schwitzer, and Jim Wright.

Whether they know it or not, the people who really do the heavy lifting on screening are taxpayers, who fund the U.S. Preventive Services Task Force and the Canadian equivalent, the Canadian Task Force on Preventive Health Care. Many of the large important screening trials carried out by the National Institutes of Health and the Canadian Institutes of Health Research are like lifelines, bringing science to the rescue of health policy around the world.

And lastly, I'd like to thank my family, Joey, Lynda, Chase, Morgan, Earla, Bruce, and Leigh-Ann, without whose love and support I'd never attempt a project like this book.

My editor, Catherine Plear, has worked an enormous amount of magic on this manuscript, but any errors in the text are mine and mine alone.

INDEX